Shared Care for Prostatic Diseases

Roger Kirby MA MD FRCS(Urol) FEBU
Consultant Urologist, St Bartholomew's Hospital, London, UK

John Fitzpatrick MCh FRCSI FEBU
Professor of Surgery, University College, Dublin, Ireland

Michael Kirby MB BS LRCP MRCS MRCP
Family Practitioner, The Surgery, Nevells Road, Letchworth, UK

Andrew Fitzpatrick MB BCh MRCGP DCH DObst (RCPI)
Family Practitioner, Peel View Medical Centre, Kirkintilloch,
Glasgow, UK

Forewords by
Louis J Denis MD FACS and **E Darracott Vaughan Jr** MD

Illustrated by
Dee McLean

Supported by an educational grant from
INVICTA™ Pharmaceuticals, a division of Pfizer Limited

I
M M
M

© 1994 Isis Medical Media Ltd
Saxon Beck, 58 St Aldates
Oxford OX1 1ST, UK

First published 1994
Reprinted 1995

British Library Cataloguing in Publication Data
A catalogue record for this title is available from the British Library

ISBN 1 899066 00 4

Library of Congress
Cataloguing-in-Publication Data

Kirby, R. (Roger)
Shared Care for Prostatic Diseases/
Roger Kirby, John Fitzpatrick, Michael Kirby, Andrew Fitzpatrick

Always refer to the manufacturer's Prescribing Information before prescribing
drugs cited in this book.

Editorial direction and project management
Sarah Redston BSc

Design and production
Design Online Ltd, Standingford House, Cave Street, Oxford OX4 1BA, UK

Printed by
Dah Hua Printing Press Co. Ltd, Hong Kong

Distributors
Times Mirror International Publishers, Medway City Estate, Rochester, Kent ME2 4DU

"Procul, o procul este, profani."

"Hence, o hence... ye that are uninitiated."

Virgil. *Aeneid;* vi, 258.

Forthcoming titles in the
Shared Care series include:

- Gastroenterology

- Gynaecology

- Asthma and allergies

Contents

Glossary

BPH	Benign prostatic hyperplasia
DES	Diethylstilboestrol
DHT	Dihydrotestosterone
DRE	Digital rectal examination
EGF	Epidermal growth factor
ELAP	Endoscopic laser ablation of the prostate
EPS	Expressed prostatic secretions
FGF	Fibroblast growth factor
FSH	Follicle stimulating hormone
HIFU	High-intensity focused ultrasound
IPSS	International Prostate Symptom Score
IVU	Intravenous urography
LH	Luteinizing hormone
LHRH	Luteinizing hormone releasing hormone
MSU	Mid-stream urine
PIN	Prostatic intra-epithelial neoplasia
PSA	Prostate-specific antigen
PVR	Post-void residual
SHBG	Sex hormone binding globulin
TGF	Transforming growth factor
TRUS	Transrectal ultrasound
TUIP	Transurethral incision of the prostate
TULIP	Transurethral laser incision of the prostate
TUMT	Transurethral microwave thermotherapy
TUNA	Transurethral needle ablation
TURP	Transurethral resection of the prostate
U&E	Urea and electrolytes
UTI	Urinary tract infection

Forewords

The collaboration between two urologists and their brothers who are family practitioners has led to this timely book on shared care for prostatic diseases. Few of the many books and articles on prostatic diseases match the vivid style, clear presentation and balanced conclusions of this work – it provides practical science, wrapped in an entertaining and thought-provoking style.

Shared Care for Prostatic Diseases addresses a controversial issue, which should be neither controversial or even an issue. The increase in the ageing populations in the industrialized world have and will continue to change the demography of disease, and the population over 60 years of age is projected to double in the next generation. In addition to this, our new senior citizens have higher expectations of quality of life than previous generations, and men in their later years with voiding problems are becoming increasingly inclined to present to their doctor in the hope of obtaining relief rather than suffer in silence.

Various scientific studies and two successful international meetings have now led to a consensus for diagnosing and managing benign prostatic hyperplasia (BPH) – the International Prostate Symptom Score (IPSS) is perhaps one of the most useful tools to have emerged. This consensus is supported by most international and national urological associations and was developed under the auspices of the World Health Organization (WHO). One of the major agreements of this consensus was that the indications for surgery were clear in only one-fifth of all patients suffering from clinical BPH. This, of course, leaves four-fifths of all patients with an option for treatments other than surgery.

In response to this need, two different medical treatments have been developed, the 5-alpha-reductase inhibitors, which reduce the volume of the adenoma, and the alpha-adrenergic-blockers, which reduce outflow resistance by relaxing the smooth muscle of the prostate. In addition, a myriad of minimally invasive procedures has been spawned, which aimed to match the positive symptomatic effects of surgery, but more efficiently and with fewer complications.

These advances have, however, created the problem of how to care for the increasing numbers of middle-aged and elderly men with voiding problems that clearly do not need surgical treatment. Shared care may be the answer, as this is exactly the cohort of patients that will benefit from the diagnosis and treatment of the early symptoms of BPH by family practitioners. *Shared Care for Prostatic Diseases* presents the practical information that family practitioners need to select patients who require prompt referral for specialist evaluation, as well as to avoid a missed diagnosis of early clinical prostate cancer.

It was the 17th century, social poet, Brederode, who preached that "one who voids in his boots will soon lose all his other attributes". Many men today still view prostate problems as the beginning of the end. We in the medical profession are, however, aware of the considerable advances that have already been made and will continue to be made in treatments for prostatic disease. A well-organized collaboration between family practitioners and urologists is the next step forward, a process for which this book is an ideal catalyst.

Louis J Denis MD FACS
Antwerp, Belgium

Undoubtedly, *Shared Care for Prostatic Diseases* is one of the first of many forthcoming books that will integrate information for primary care physicians and specialists working together to improve patient care. We are entering an era which will focus more on society's interest in health than on complex treatments for disease. In addition, the role of primary care physicians will gain further emphasis as we attempt to reduce healthcare costs.

Shared Care for Prostatic Diseases does an excellent job in presenting a well-organized, current and comprehensive, but readable, account of the management of patients with prostatic diseases. Oriented primarily for the primary care physician, the book also contains pertinent information for the urologist. As the authors articulate, we are fortunate in having developed patient questionnaires that quantify the symptoms of BPH, give an index of the impact of the disease on their quality of life, and form part of the recently developed clinical care guidelines. The important aspect of these patient-derived indices is that they standardize our approach to patients, simplifying the job of primary care physicians for whom treating patients with prostatic disease is only one small part of their day-to-day activities.

It is appropriate that this book presents in detail the current guidelines for the diagnosis and care of patients with BPH and prostatic cancer. This background information sets the framework for deciding when to refer the patient to the urologist for further evaluation and/or treatment. While areas of controversy remain, the concepts delivered in the initial chapters of the book are current and lend themselves to modifications as our knowledge increases.

The later chapters discuss the current medical and surgical treatments of patients with BPH and prostatic cancer. I like to think of the treatment of patients with BPH as 'step therapy'. Initially, patients with low symptom scores are managed with 'watchful waiting' and periodic evaluation. As their symptoms increase and their quality of life is adversely affected, patients can be started on medical therapy.

If these modalities fail to correct the underlying abnormalities and relieve the symptoms, patients are candidates for evolving 'intermediate' therapies, including laser treatment, thermotherapy or high-intensity focused ultrasound. Finally, if 'intermediate' therapies are ineffective, the 'gold standard' of transurethral prostatectomy or open prostatectomy is utilized. It should be remembered that some patients desire intervention early in the course of their disease so as to have the best chance of eliminating disturbing symptoms.

The management of prostate cancer is less clear, but the controversies are concisely outlined in the text. At present, the general thought is that patients with localized disease should be identified with appropriate studies and treated for cure with either total prostatectomy or external beam irradiation. The treatment decision is obviously age-dependent and there is probably a subset of patients over the age of 70 years with well-differentiated tumours that can be observed without treatment. The alternatives for treatment of patients with metastatic disease are outlined and recommendations given, though it is emphasized that management of these patients will undoubtedly change in the near future.

The case studies at the end are used to illustrate specific situations and enhance the overall effectiveness of the information given, allowing the reader to put into practice the information gained from the book as a whole.

Shared care is clearly the way forward for managing patients with prostatic disease, and a great deal of responsibility is going to be placed on the primary care physician. It is the role of the specialists, the urologists, who spend much time thinking about these diseases, to communicate our current knowledge to the primary care physician. This task has been addressed with great care and thought by the authors, and the result will be of benefit to primary care physicians, urologists and, most importantly, patients with these diseases.

E Darracott Vaughan Jr MD
New York, USA

Preface

A Cinderella subject for many years, the prostate has recently become the focus of intense medical and public interest. The tremendous advances made in the development of new, effective drugs and less invasive therapies has meant that there are now real options for the treatment of prostatic diseases other than surgery. This progress, together with a heightened awareness of the considerable prevalence of these diseases, has been reflected in the media which, almost weekly, seem to feature some aspect of prostatic disease.

As the expectations of our ever-swelling ranks of middle-aged and elderly populations increase, men with prostate problems are presenting to us in greater and greater numbers. Shared care for prostatic disease will enable family practitioners and urologists to provide these men with the best quality and most cost-effective care possible. As the first port of call, the family practitioner's role is crucial. However, only by working in close cooperation with the urologist can the decision as to whether to reassure the patient, commence medical therapy or refer for medical evaluation be made with accuracy and confidence.

In producing this book, two urologists and their brothers who are family practitioners have worked with Dee McLean, a leading medical artist, to provide a comprehensive, but readily readable account of the prostate which is applicable to clinical practice. We hope that this book will be widely read by all those with an interest in caring for the ever-increasing number of men whose quality of life is affected by prostate problems.

RSK, JMF, MGK, APF

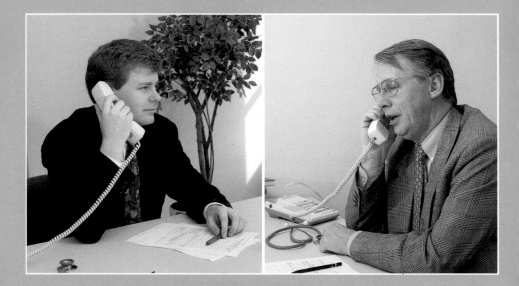

Chapter 1

The shared care concept

Shared care for prostatic disease is the joint management of men with prostate problems by family practitioners and urologists. Like many new ideas, this concept has been born out of necessity to manage change constructively. Traditionally, the diagnosis and management of prostatic disorders has largely been handled by urologists for whom there was usually a relatively simple decision – to operate or not to operate. Two recent developments, in particular, have conspired to challenge the *modus operandi*.

- Epidemiological surveys have suggested that mild-to-moderate symptoms of benign prostatic hyperplasia (BPH) are extremely prevalent in men who never seek the advice of a urologist[1].
- The availability of new treatment options for BPH have made men reluctant to accept transurethral resection of the prostate (TURP) as the first-line therapy, favouring medical and less invasive alternatives instead.

Quality of life

Disorders of the prostate are a major source of discomfort and disease in middle-aged and elderly men. Almost half of all men over the age of 65 suffer some symptoms of bladder outflow obstruction due to BPH[1,2], which often significantly reduce their quality of life[3,4]. Furthermore, prostate cancer is now the second commonest cause of cancer death in men in many countries.

Over the coming years, family practitioners and urologists alike

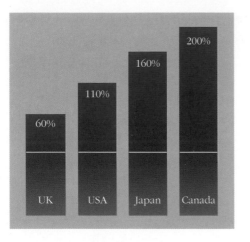

Figure 1.1 *Projected percentage increase in population over 60 years of age by the year 2020. As the world's population ages, a dramatic increase in the number of patients presenting with prostate problems is expected.*

will see a dramatic increase in the number of patients presenting with prostate problems. One important reason for this is the continuing rise in the proportion of the world's population over the age of 60 (Figure 1.1)[5]. Another reason is the increasing public awareness that the bothersome symptoms of BPH can now be treated with either new medical therapies or minimally invasive, short-stay surgery rather than procedures requiring hospital admission and anaesthesia. Based on recent epidemiological data, in Europe, for example, to submit all those men over the age of 60 whose quality of life is negatively affected by the symptoms of BPH to surgery would mean increasing the current TURP rate more than 10-fold and radically increasing the number of fully trained urologists[4].

Attitudes towards prostate cancer are also changing. Men in their so-called 'third age' (50–75 years) no longer consider themselves old, and are less prepared to accept reduced quality of life due to waning health and increasing cancer risk as an inevitable accompaniment to the passage of time. Earlier diagnosis and improved methods of treatment are now commonly featured in the media, and men are beginning to press their doctors for a 'prostate health check'. Prostate disease will therefore have an increasing impact on health economics[6], which raises the question – how can these patients best be managed?

Shared care – meeting the need for treatment

The challenge is to evolve a strategy that permits those patients with the most need of more specialist evaluation and intervention (e.g. men under 75 years with significant volume prostate cancer or those with severely obstructive BPH) rapid access to diagnosis and treatment by urologists. By contrast, those with only minor symptoms and no evidence of coexistent prostate cancer, who were formerly candidates for 'watchful waiting' in urology clinics, can be cared for by appropriately informed and educated family practitioners. This process has been termed 'shared care'.

Advantages of a shared-care approach

The overall benefit of shared care for prostatic disease is improved patient care. However, its advantages to all those involved can be significant (Table 1.1). Indeed, far from reducing the diagnosis of prostate cancer, the introduction of shared care and medical therapy should increase the detection of early potentially curable lesions. Furthermore, in these times of increasing budgetary restrictions in most healthcare systems, a shared-care approach is likely to be cost-effective and therefore encouraged by the governments and insurance companies who hold the purse-strings.

Raising awareness

The key to advancing this concept of shared care is to raise awareness of the prevalence and importance of both BPH and prostate cancer, not only among the general public, but also among family practitioners. Recent population-based surveys have shown a lamentably low level of public knowledge relating to the prostate[7]. Family practitioners also often seem somewhat bewildered by the diseases afflicting this organ: a recent survey of family practitioners in London, UK revealed that the great majority performed less than five digital rectal examinations (DRE) a month[8]. This strongly suggests that middle-aged and elderly men whose quality of life is being affected adversely by prostatic disease, ascribe the symptoms to ageing, and do not trouble their

Table 1.1 Advantages of a shared-care approach for prostatic diseases

Patients
- Reduced hospital visits and waiting times
- Easier access to local medical advice
- Greater continuity of treatment and better follow-up
- Greater contact with the family practitioner, who is more aware of their medical/social history

Family practitioners
- Patients may be more open with healthcare professionals with whom they are familiar
- Opportunity for family practitioners to broaden their knowledge of prostatic disease and develop new skills
- Rewards of team working and providing better patient care

Urologists
- Reduced hospital admissions and surgical waiting times
- Encourages more appropriate referrals
- Earlier diagnosis of prostate cancer
- More time available for patients requiring specialist management
- Rewards of stronger relations with community physicians and providing better patient care

family practitioner. Furthermore, the prostate seldom attracts specific enquiry in most standard health checks (Figure 1.2). The result – problems remain neglected, underdiagnosed and untreated.

Prostate disease – the three questions
In fact, the first step in detecting prostate disease, which is very simple for a family practitioner to undertake at a routine visit, is asking the so-called 'three questions'.

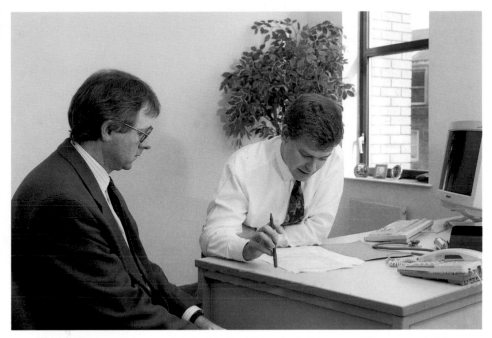

Figure 1.2 *Enquiries into prostate health should form part of the general fitness appraisal for middle-aged and elderly men.*

■ Do you get up at night to pass urine?
■ Is your urinary stream reduced?
■ Are you bothered by bladder symptoms ('your waterworks')?

Most afflicted patients will give an affirmative to at least two of the three questions, and then the severity of the problem can be quantified by asking the patient to complete an International Prostate Symptom Score (IPSS) sheet (see page 54).

The logistics of shared care

As family practitioners have become more conversant with the management of the specific disease processes, such as uncomplicated diabetes, asthma, hypertension and lipid disorders, they have become more expert in selecting those cases most appropriate for specialist referral. This process has been supported by educational back-up from the specialists involved. Similar support will also be necessary when considering the logistics of moving towards a shared-care approach for managing patients with prostate problems.

In the light of recent advances, family practitioners will probably need to update and expand their knowledge and skills in the treatment of prostate disease (Figure 1.3), and local urologists must be prepared to provide the relevant help, information and, if necessary, tuition (Figure 1.4). This learning curve can only be climbed by the interaction and cooperation of urologists and their referring family practitioners.

Ultimate goal

It must be remembered that BPH is a multifactorial disease with varied manifestations, and that prostatic cancer may masquerade as, or coexist with, BPH. In this book, we shall consider to what extent

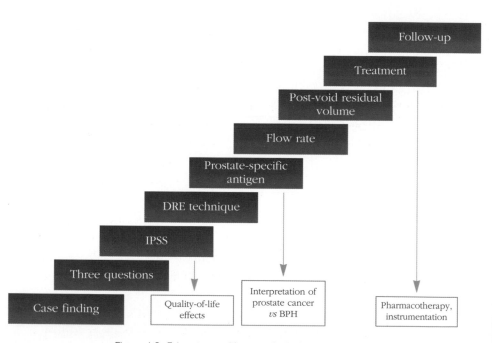

Figure 1.3. *Education and how to climb the learning steps.*

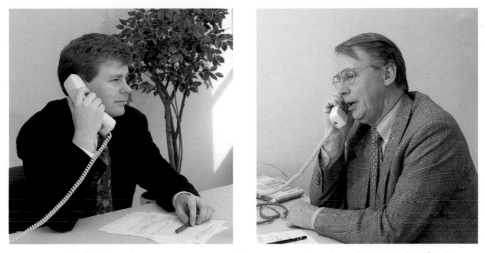

Figure 1.4 *Feedback from the urologist is invaluable, especially in the early stages when family practitioners are learning new diagnosis and management procedures.*

prostate disorders may safely be handled by the family practitioner, and attempt to identify those patients who should be referred promptly for specialist evaluation, and perhaps surgery, by a urologist.

The ultimate goal of 'shared care' for prostatic disorders is to enhance patient care both by improving understanding of these diseases, and by fostering closer links between family practitioners and urologists. The rewards of these endeavours may be considerable. Family practitioners will gain satisfaction from improved patient management within their practices, and reduced time and money spent on inappropriate referrals; and, in turn, urologists will be able to dedicate more effort to those patients in whom specific urological intervention can make a significant impact on the extent and quality of their life. Most important of all, patients themselves will benefit from an increasingly more efficient and appropriate referral and treatment pattern.

It is appreciated that healthcare provision varies greatly from country to country in terms of the ratios of urologists:family practitioners and the relationships between them. The number of

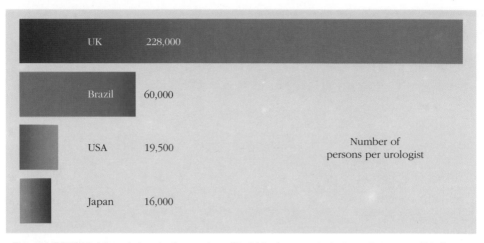

Figure 1.5 *Worldwide variations in the number of individuals per urologist in each country will influence the development of shared care for prostatic disease in different countries.*

urologists per capita also varies widely (Figure 1.5). This book will therefore concentrate on the overriding general principles of patient management, rather than country-specific details. However, the final chapter comprises a comprehensive set of case histories showing shared care 'in action'.

Summary

- Many middle-aged and elderly men suffer symptoms of prostate disease that adversely affect their quality of life and yet go untreated.

- The traditional role of urologists handling all patients with prostate disorders may no longer be appropriate due to an increasingly elderly population and the introduction of effective medical treatments.

- Family practitioners and urologists can work together to improve patient care; this is the 'shared care' concept.

■ Clinical BPH may be revealed by asking three questions and quantified by a formal symptom score (e.g. the IPSS).

■ Shared care should increase rather than decrease the early diagnosis of prostate cancer.

References

1 Garraway WM, Collins GN, Lee RJ. High prevalence of benign prostatic hypertrophy in the community. *Lancet* 1991; **338**: 469–71.

2 Chute CG, Panser LA, Girman CJ *et al.* The prevalence of prostatism: a population-based survey of urinary symptoms. *J Urol* 1993; **150**: 85–9.

3 Tsang KT, Garraway WM. Impact of benign prostatic hyperplasia on general well-being of men. *Prostate* 1993; **23**: 1–7.

4 Garraway WM, Russell EBAW, Lee RJ *et al.* Impact of previously unrecognised benign prostatic hyperplasia on daily activities of middle-aged and elderly men. *Br J Gen Pract* 1993; **43**: 318–21.

5 Brody JA. Prospects of an ageing population. *Nature* 1985; **315**: 463–6.

6 Duncan BM, Garraway WM. Prostatic surgery for benign prostatic hyperplasia: meeting the expanding demand. *Br J Urol* 1993; **72**: 761–5.

7 Boyle P, Cox B, Macfarlane GJ, Matillon Y, Kell U, La Vecchia C. Knowledge and attitudes of men in France, Italy, the United Kingdom and Germany to the prostate and symptoms of its diseases. *Euro J Public Health* 1994 (in press).

8 Hennigan TW, Franks PJ, Hocken DB, Allen-Mersh TG. Rectal examination in general practice. *BMJ* 1990; **301**: 478–80.

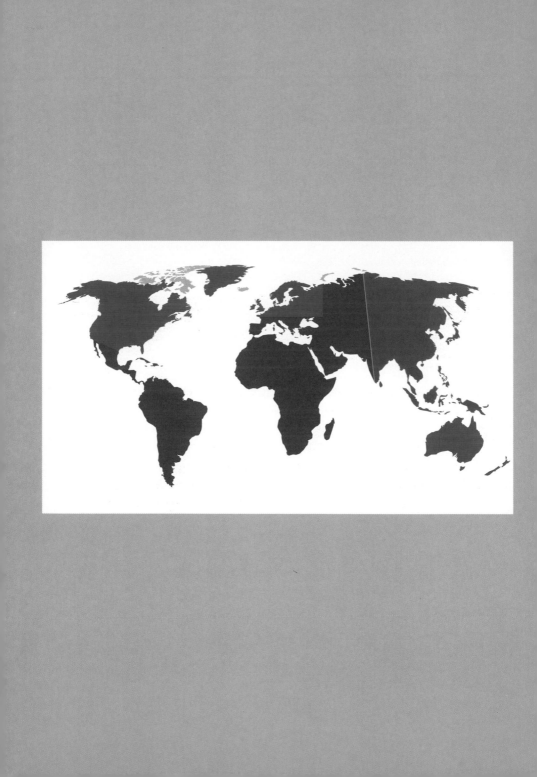

Chapter 2

Extent of the problem

Worldwide, demographic shifts are leading towards an increasingly aged society and, as a result, the absolute numbers of patients being diagnosed with benign prostatic hyperplasia (BPH) and subsequently requiring therapy for prostatic disease will continue to rise[1]. By the year 2000, the life expectancy of males at birth will exceed 80 years in many countries, and most men can therefore be expected to live to an age at which they have an 88% chance of developing histological BPH and more than a 50% chance of symptomatic BPH. In addition to this, clinical prostate cancer seems set to reach epidemic proportions in the next 25 years, perhaps trebling by the year 2020[1]. A major effort is therefore required to lessen the impact of these prostatic diseases on our increasingly long-lived population.

The three most common diseases affecting the prostate, in decreasing order, are BPH, prostate cancer and prostatitis (Figure 2.1).

Epidemiology of BPH

Although millions of men suffer from BPH, published natural history studies have unfortunately involved only a few hundred patients. In discussing the epidemiology and natural history of BPH, it is necessary to distinguish:

■ histological BPH, usually determined on autopsy findings
■ clinical BPH indicated by an enlarged prostate on digital rectal examination (DRE) or visible by imaging studies, such as transrectal ultrasound (TRUS)

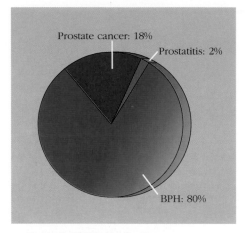

Figure 2.1 *BPH is by far the most common condition in men presenting with prostate problems.*

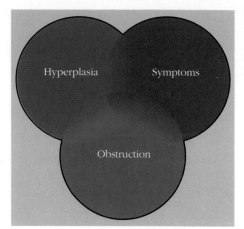

Figure 2.2 *The three fundamental features of BPH – hyperplasia, symptoms and obstruction – may occur independently or may coexist.*

■ the symptoms of BPH usually referred to as 'prostatism'.

As illustrated in the overlapping circles of Figure 2.2, prostatic enlargement due to BPH, symptoms of 'prostatism' and outflow obstruction may occur independently or coexist.

Prevalence of BPH

The prevalence of histological, clinical and symptomatic BPH all increase with age. This association with ageing may reflect an age-related hormonal imbalance between testosterone and oestrogens (see Chapter 4).

Autopsy studies[2] have shown that the prevalence of histological BPH appears to rise from around 50% in men in their 60s to 90% in men over 85 years of age. The proportion of men with palpable prostatic enlargement, however, is rather less, with a prevalence of 21% in men aged between 50 and 60 years, rising to approximately 53% in men in their 80s.

Most important, of course, is the proportion of men who are troubled by symptoms. Data from the Baltimore Longitudinal Study of Ageing suggest that the prevalence of symptomatic BPH is around

14% in men in their 40s, 24% in men in their 50s, and 43% in men beyond the age of 60 (Figure 2.3)[3]. These data highlight the fact that the presence of either histological evidence of BPH or palpable enlargement of the gland is not always associated with clinically significant bladder outflow obstruction.

Hidden prevalence. A recent population-based study from Stirling, UK also reported a prevalence of symptomatic BPH of 43% in men over 60[4]. About half of the men with

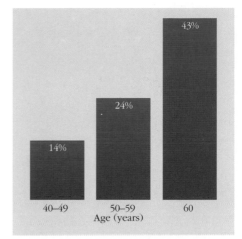

Figure 2.3 *The prevalence of symptomatic BPH increases with age; almost half the men over 60 years of age are affected.*

evidence of obstructive BPH (defined as a prostate on TRUS > 20 g, and symptoms of urinary dysfunction and/or a peak urine flow rate of < 15 ml/second) reported interference with one or more activities of daily living (Table 2.1, Figure 2.4), compared with 28% of men without the condition. In addition to this quality-of-life impairment,

Table 2.1 Adverse effects of the symptoms of BPH on activities of daily living

- Limits fluid intake before travel
- Restricts fluid intake before bedtime
- Cannot drive for 2 hours without a break
- Disruption of sleep
- Limits going to places without toilets
- Limits playing outdoor sports
- Avoids, for example, going to cinema, theatre or church

many patients reported worry and embarrassment about their urinary function[5].

Another study found that the irritative symptoms (i.e. frequency, urgency and nocturia) were more 'bothersome' and had more impact on quality of life than the obstructive symptoms (i.e. hesitancy, poor stream and post-micturition dribbling)[6]. Despite this measurable effect on quality of life, very few of these individuals had in fact consulted their doctor about their symptoms.

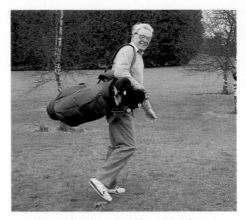

Figure 2.4 *Quality of life – a significant proportion of men with symptomatic BPH avoid sport and leisure activities because of their symptoms.*

A Danish study has also recorded the reluctance among men aged 60–79 to consult a doctor about prostatic symptoms[7]. Why they do not seek medical help remains unclear, but some of the most likely reasons are shown in Table 2.2. Clearly, there is scope for improving both the level of public education and the knowledge of healthcare professionals in this area.

Effects of race and environment

Although worldwide variations in the prevalence of BPH have been reported, wide disparities in life expectancy may account for some of these differences. Clinical as opposed to histological BPH may be more common among black races, but further studies are needed to verify this[8]. Inherited factors have, however, been implicated to explain the high rates of symptomatic BPH reported from the central and northern parts of the Sudan, where intermarriage has often occurred between Arabs and indigenous Africans, whereas no cases were found in the pure African populations of the Southern Sudan[9]. Also in New Orleans, USA, it has been shown that a higher prevalence of clinical BPH occurs in blacks than whites[10].

Table 2.2 Reasons why men with symptoms of prostatic disease do not present to their doctor

■ Perception that symptoms are a normal feature of ageing
■ Fear of a diagnosis of cancer
■ Fear of surgery and its potential side-effects
■ Reluctance to discuss symptoms with a female family practitioner
■ Fear of ridicule, and embarrassment of discussing symptoms
■ Dislike of digital rectal examination
■ Reluctance to travel long distances from home for diagnosis and treatment

By contrast, clinical BPH seems relatively rare in the Far East. In 1900 autopsies performed in Peking (now Beijing) over a period of 41 years, the incidence of histological BPH was found to be only 6.6% among the native Chinese and 47.2% in other ethnic groups[11]. The suggestion that South-East Asians who migrate to the USA acquire a higher rate of BPH than their counterparts remaining in South-East Asia, points to an environmental and dietary influence.

Dietary factors
A study from Japan has shown that the incidence of BPH is higher in men consuming large amounts of milk than in those with a high vegetable intake. It has been postulated that certain yellow vegetables and other elements in the Japanese diet, including soya, which are known to contain phyto-oestrogens may exert some protective effect against the development of BPH[12].

Associated conditions
It has also been proposed, but without much corroborative evidence, that BPH is more likely to develop in patients with diabetes mellitus, hypertension and cardiovascular disease[13]. Conversely, cirrhosis of the

liver may be associated with a lower incidence of BPH. Theoretically, this could be due to changes in steroid metabolism leading to a relative increase in oestrogen and sex hormone binding globulin (SHBG), which may in turn protect the prostatic stroma from the stimulatory effects of androgens[14].

Epidemiology of prostate cancer

Increasing prevalence

Prostate cancer is an important public health problem which also seems set to increase. A quarter of a million cases were diagnosed worldwide in 1980, of which 85,000 new cases were in Europe. In Europe and North America, prostate cancer is the second most lethal malignancy in men after lung cancer, and now accounts for one in ten of all cancer deaths in men in many developed countries. As with BPH, prostate cancer seems certain to increase in absolute terms simply because of the ageing population.

Effects of race

Although few studies have researched the epidemiology of prostate cancer, some facts are known. The incidence of clinical prostate cancer varies widely throughout the world, with the highest rates being seen in north-west Europe and North America, the lowest rates in Eastern Asia and moderate rates in Africa (Figure 2.5). Data from Africa are, however, unreliable and life expectancy is low, and this may lead to serious under-estimation. Interestingly, the incidence is much higher in areas with a population of African descent, such as the Caribbean and north-east Brazil[15].

In the USA, there is a well-documented increased risk of prostate cancer in blacks compared with whites. Blacks also appear prone to develop the disease earlier and, perhaps, in a more aggressive form, and therefore have a higher mortality from the disease[16]. Although the reasons for this are not entirely clear, the higher incidence of prostate cancer in blacks may partly be due to the lower age of first sexual intercourse and the higher number of sexual partners, both of which are thought to be associated with a higher risk of prostate cancer.

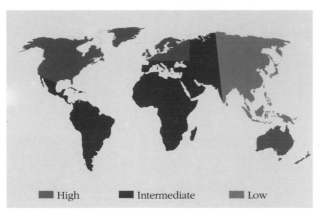

High   Intermediate   Low

Figure 2.5 *Relative incidences of prostate cancer in different countries.*

Japanese men appear to have reduced 5-alpha-reductase activity in the prostate gland which may protect them from developing cancer. The converse is true in American blacks[17]. Thus differences in androgen metabolism could account for the varying susceptibilities to this disease.

Effects of diet

Migration from Japan to the USA leads to a 15–20-fold increase in the incidence of prostate cancer. Dramatic increases occur in the first and second generations and then level out to match the high prevalence rates of prostate cancer found in Americans. This effect may be related to diet, and this theory is supported by the observation of an increasing tendency to adopt a more 'western' diet. An increased fat and red meat consumption may have a positive effect on the incidence of prostate cancer, as it has on other diseases.

Other factors

Occupational risk. The risk of prostate cancer may be increased in men who work with cadmium or in the nuclear power industry[18].

Vasectomy. Although several case-controlled studies have suggested a link between vasectomy and prostate cancer[19], closer scrutiny of these data has cast doubt on this contention[20]. Currently patients can be reassured that there is little evidence of a definite link.

Genetic predisposition. Recently, the possibility of a genetic predisposition towards prostate cancer in some families has been proposed[21]. Individuals with a first-degree relative with prostate cancer diagnosed at a young age have been estimated to have a 2.2 increased relative risk of developing the disease themselves; those with two first-degree relatives affected have more than twice this risk.

Summary

■ BPH is the most prevalent disease to affect men beyond middle age.

■ Although clinical BPH is associated with significant impairment of quality of life, many BPH sufferers are reluctant to consult a doctor, perhaps because of fear of surgery or cancer.

■ Prostate cancer is now the second most common cause of cancer death in men.

■ As the population of the world progressively ages, so the burden of BPH and prostate cancer will inevitably rise.

References

1   Carter HB, Coffey DS. The prostate: an increasing medical problem. *Prostate* 1990; **16**: 39–48.

2   Guess HA, Arrighi HM, Metter ET, Fozard JL. Cumulative prevalence of prostatism matches the autopsy prevalence of benign prostatic hyperplasia. *Prostate* 1990; **17**: 214–46.

3   Berry SJ, Coffey DS, Walsh PC, Ewing LL. The development of human benign prostatic hyperplasia with age. *J Urol* 1984; **132**: 474–9.

4   Garraway WM, Collins GN, Lee RJ. High prevalence of benign prostatic hypertrophy in the community. *Lancet* 1991; **338**: 469–71.

5   Garraway WM, McKelvie GB, Russell EBAW *et al.* Impact of previously unrecognised benign prostatic hyperplasia on the daily activities of middle-aged and elderly men. *Br J Gen Pract* 1993; **43**: 318–21.

6   Department of Veterans Affairs cooperative study of transurethral resection for benign prostatic hyperplasia. A comparison of quality of life with patient reported symptoms and objective findings in men with benign prostatic hyperplasia. *J Urol* 1993; **150**: 1696–1700.

7   Sommer P, Nielson KK, Bauer T. Voiding patterns in men evaluated by a questionnaire survey. *Br J Urol* 1990; **65**: 155–60.

8   Rotkin ID. Origins, distribution, and risk of benign prostatic hypertrophy. In: Hinman F, Boyarsky S, eds. *Benign Prostatic Hypertrophy*. New York: Springer-Verlag, 1983: 10–21.

9   Kambal A. Prostatic obstruction in Sudan. *Br J Urol* 1977; **49**: 139–41.

10   Derbes VDP, Leche SM, Hooker CW. The incidence of benign prostatic hypertrophy among the whites and negroes in New Orleans. *J Urol* 1937; **38**: 383–8.

11   Chang HL, Chan CY. Benign hypertrophy of the prostate. *Chin Med J* 1936; **50**: 1707–22.

12   Araki H, Watanabe H, Mishina T, Nakao M. High-risk group for benign prostatic hypertrophy. *Prostate* 1983; **4**: 253–64.

13   Bourke JB, Griffin JP. Diabetes mellitus in patients with prostatic hyperplasia. *BMJ* 1968; **4**: 492–3.

14   Robson MC. The incidence of benign prostatic hyperplasia and prostatic carcinoma in cirrhosis of the liver. *J Urol* 1964; **92**: 307–10.

15   Wilson JMG. Epidemiology of prostate cancer. In: Bruce AW, Trachtenberg J, eds. *Adenocarcinoma of the prostate*. London: Springer-Verlag, 1987: 1–28.

16   Levine RL, Wilchinsky M. Adenocarcinoma of the prostate: a comparison of the disease in blacks versus whites. *J Urol* 1979; **121**: 761–2.

17   Ross HK, Bernstein L, Lobow RA, Khimizu H, Stanezyk FC, Pike MC, 5 alpha reductase activity and the risk of prostate cancer among Japanese and US white and black males. *Lancet* 1992; **339**: 887–9.

18   Rooney C, Beral V, Maconochie N, Fraser P, Davies G. Case-control study of prostatic cancer in employees of the United Kindgom Atomic Energy Authority. *BMJ* 1993; **307**: 1391–7.

19   Rosenberg L, Palmer JR, Zeba AG, Warshauer ME, Stolley PD, Shapiro S. Vasectomy and the risk of prostate cancer. *Am J Epidemiol* 1990; **132**: 1051–5.

20   Editorial: Vasectomy and prostate cancer. *Lancet* 1991; **337**: 1445–6.

21   Steinberg GN, Carter BS, Beaty TH, Childs B, Walsh PC. Family history and the risk of prostate cancer. *The Prostate* 1990; **17**: 337–47.

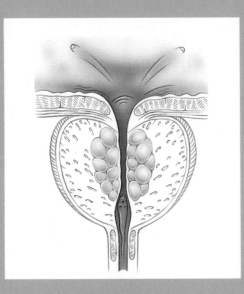

Chapter 3

Development of prostatic disease

Since antiquity, benign prostatic hyperplasia (BPH) has been recognized as a condition that affects men beyond middle age. Although Hippocrates was probably referring to BPH when he wrote that "disorders of the bladder are difficult to treat in older men", the first true description of the gland was by Herophilus of Alexandria.

In 1788, John Hunter noted that the prostate depended on testicular function for normal growth, and he also described the consequences of bladder outflow obstruction due to prostatic enlargement (Figure 3.1).

The three zones of the prostate

Almost 200 years later, McNeal[1] demonstrated that the prostate gland is divided into two morphologically distinct zones, central and peripheral, that comprise 25% and 70% of the normal prostatic volume,

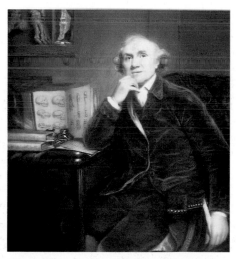

Figure 3.1 *John Hunter (1728–1793), one of the fathers of surgery, discovered that prostate growth is a hormone-dependent process.*

Figure 3.2 *Anatomy and morphology of the prostate. BPH develops in the transition zone while cancer more commonly commences in the peripheral zone.*

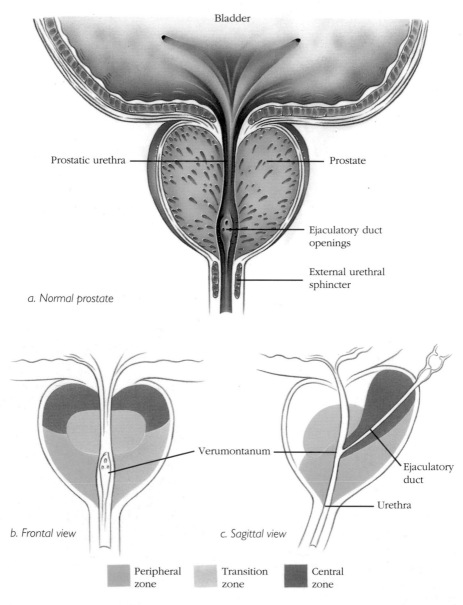

Bladder

Prostatic urethra

Prostate

Ejaculatory duct openings

External urethral sphincter

a. Normal prostate

Verumontanum

Ejaculatory duct

Urethra

b. Frontal view

c. Sagittal view

Peripheral zone

Transition zone

Central zone

respectively (Figure 3.2). The remaining 5% of the normal gland consists of the transition zone, which lies adjacent to the urethra and extends up to the bladder neck.

Although the histological characteristics of the transition zone and the peripheral zone are similar, the transition zone is the site of development of BPH, while the adjacent peripheral zone is prone to the development of cancer.

Natural history of BPH

Obstruction due to BPH is thought to be gradually progressive, resulting eventually in either acute or chronic urinary retention. However, in a study of 107 men with mild prostatism, only 10 men required surgery and the remaining 97 showed little objective evidence of worsening obstruction[2]. This view is supported by a family practice-based study reported in 1969[3], which found that of 60 patients with moderate symptoms of prostatism not immediately subjected to surgery, 48% had no urinary symptoms at final follow-up, 4–7 years later. Other authors have noted that the symptoms of prostatic obstruction may naturally wax and wane (Figure 3.3)[4]. In an ongoing study by the Veterans Administration in the USA, patients with BPH have been randomized to 'watchful waiting' *versus* immediate transurethral resection of the prostate (TURP). It is now emerging that the 'watchful waiting' group, especially those with mild-to-moderate symptoms, appear to do quite well during follow-up, although the reduction in symptom score is rather less than that in the operated group.

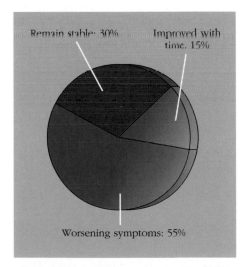

Figure 3.3 *Natural history of symptoms of BPH.*

23

Slow progression

Overall, however, there is probably a very slow progression in most cases of clinical BPH. Longitudinal population-based studies have demonstrated a mean annual decline of maximum flow rate of around 0.2 ml/second[5]; although this probably mainly reflects the effect of slowly developing prostatic enlargement, it has to be conceded that a gradual decline in detrusor contractility related to age may also be a contributory factor[6].

Pathology of BPH

Appearance of microscopic stromal nodules

The first changes of BPH, which may begin around the age of 40, consist of microscopic stromal nodules that occur in the transition zone around the periurethral area; glandular hyperplasia begins around these small nodules. The nodules may vary in size from a few millimetres to a few centimetres, and are composed of either glandular elements, fibromuscular elements (stroma) or a mixture of both; the smooth muscle containing stroma is generally by far the larger component[7]. In contrast to clinical BPH, the incidence of microscopic BPH does not vary greatly from country to country, and seems equally common in both western and developing nations, suggesting that the prevalence of microscopic BPH increases with age in all male populations.

Tissue types and obstruction

The proportion of mainly stromal (fibromuscular) nodules to mixed fibro-adenomatous nodules varies from person to person, and may help to explain why there is little correlation between prostatic size and the severity of outflow obstruction. The degree of obstruction produced by transition zone hyperplasia may reflect the proportion of smooth muscle as opposed to glandular tissue within the stroma. Prostatic smooth muscle is sympathetically innervated and its tone is subject to day-to-day and hour-to-hour neural fluctuation. This may lead to variable urethral compression. In addition, middle lobe enlargement may lead to a particularly severe ball-valve type of obstruction without much overall enlargement of the gland.

The role of PSA

The epithelial cells of BPH elaborate and secrete large quantities of prostate-specific antigen (PSA), a protease whose function it is to liquify semen after ejaculation. Low levels of PSA (< 4.0 ng/ml) are normally measurable in the serum of men. Serum PSA levels may be elevated in 25% or more of patients with BPH and in most of those with significant prostate cancer. Stamey has reported that the serum PSA value increases by an average of 0.3 ng/ml for each gram of BPH tissue present (Figure 3.4). This is only one-tenth of the increase resulting from each gram of prostate cancer tissue[8].

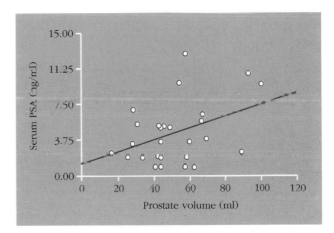

Figure 3.4 *PSA levels increase with prostatic enlargement.*

Effects of prostatic enlargement on the urinary tract

Early effects

As the development of BPH is insidious, changes within the lower urinary tract occur gradually, often making them difficult for the patient, his partner or relatives to perceive (Figure 3.5). Obstruction to urine flow results from reduced distensibility of the prostatic urethra,

Figure 3.5 *Progressive development of benign prostatic hyperplasia.*

(a) Mild BPH. This condition arises just underneath the lining of the prostatic urethra in the transition zone of the prostate.

(b) Moderate BPH. As the tissue grows, it encroaches upon and pushes into the channel of the prostatic urethra.

(c) Severe BPH. The hyperplastic tissue has replaced most of the true prostate tissue and severely restricts the channel of the prostatic urethra.

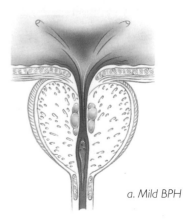

a. Mild BPH

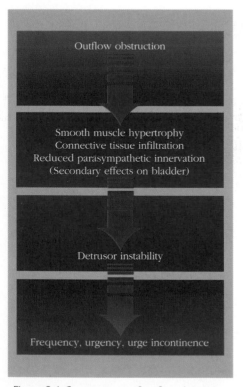

Outflow obstruction

Smooth muscle hypertrophy
Connective tissue infiltration
Reduced parasympathetic innervation
(Secondary effects on bladder)

Detrusor instability

Frequency, urgency, urge incontinence

Figure 3.6 *Consequences of outflow obstruction.*

which is caused by an enlarging prostate. This leads to a loss of bladder compliance and involuntary ('unstable') detrusor contractions during filling in up to 70% of patients[9].

As in other smooth muscle systems, the response of the detrusor to obstruction is a combination of smooth muscle cell hypertrophy and connective-tissue infiltration[10]. In addition, the density of parasympathetic nerves is significantly reduced. This leads to a relative denervation of the smooth muscle, which responds by secondary detrusor instability[11] (Figure 3.6). This denervation may explain not only the irritative symptoms of clinical

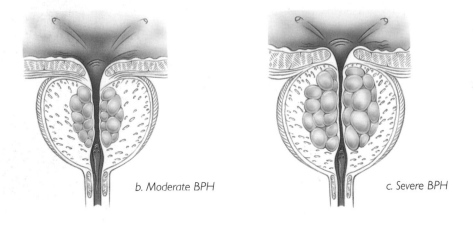

b. Moderate BPH   c. Severe BPH

BPH, but also the persistent symptoms of frequency and urgency following transurethral resection of the prostate (TURP), which may last for up to 1 year after operation. During this time, gradual reinnervation may occur, producing a progressive improvement in symptoms.

Associated pathology. Patients often tend to ignore the obstructive symptoms of prostatism, such as poor flow and hesitancy, and are more troubled as irritative symptoms develop[12]. It must be remembered, however, that these symptoms of frequency, urgency and nocturia, which have been shown to have a greater impact on quality of life, may also occur in the presence of other urinary tract pathology, such as urinary tract tuberculosis, carcinoma *in situ* or bladder stones. Urgent referral should be considered in patients with disproportionately severe symptoms, and especially haematuria.

Late effects

Chronic urinary retention. Gradual overdistension of the detrusor muscle may result in enuresis, as well as the classic symptoms of prostatism; chronic retention of urine should be considered in any elderly man who develops enuresis. When massive overdistension of the detrusor muscle occurs, the degree of denervation and associated smooth muscle damage may be so profound that full recovery of bladder function is virtually impossible.

Acute urinary retention. It is unfortunate that so many men still present with acute urinary retention without having experienced prominent BPH-related symptoms. Acute retention is a traumatic life event, and surgery for acute retention carries a higher risk of mortality and morbidity than elective TURP[13]. Severe symptoms and a large volume of residual urine are both risk factors for acute retention.

Other effects

Long-standing bladder outlet obstruction may also result in:

■ bladder stone formation

■ vesico-ureteric reflux

■ dilatation of the upper tracts with hydroureter and hydronephrosis.

Over a prolonged period, renal impairment may result and symptoms of uraemia may develop.

Other symptoms related to bladder outflow obstruction may occur including the development of bladder diverticula, urinary tract infection and pyelonephritis (Figure 3.7). Bladder calculi result in intermittent obstruction, frequency and dysuria, as well as urinary tract infection. The congested vascular bed of the prostate may sometimes lead to intermittent haematuria, which is often maximal on initiation of urination, and must be investigated to exclude coexistent transitional cell carcinoma or other malignancy.

Natural history of prostate cancer

Prostate cancer occurs only occasionally before the age of 45. However, both the incidence and mortality of prostate cancer increase with each decade, peaking at about 70 years of age[14]. Mortality from prostate cancer declines after the age of 80, but this is probably the result of competing reasons for death. In contrast, survival rates for prostate cancer observed in patients diagnosed before the age of 55 have been lower. This may be due to a more aggressive form of the disease in younger men or, possibly, later diagnosis as a result of failure to suspect the disease in this age group.

Figure 3.7 *Secondary effects of bladder outflow obstruction due to BPH.*

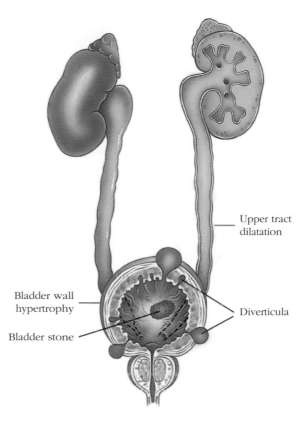

Upper tract
dilatation

Bladder wall
hypertrophy

Diverticula

Bladder stone

Pathology of prostate cancer

Careful histological studies into the pathology of prostate cancer have
revealed that:

■ 70% arise in the more glandular peripheral zone

■ 15–20% arise in the central zone

■ 10–15% arise in the transition zone.

Staging of prostate cancer

Clinical classification of prostate cancer can be achieved using the
TNM system (Table 3.1, Figure 3.8).

Table 3.1 Classification of prostate cancer

Staging

T1 – Incidental (impalpable and non-visualized by ultrasound)
T2 – Locally confined to the prostate
T3 – Locally extensive
T4 – Fixation or invasion of neighbouring organs

N0 – No regional lymph node metastasis
N1 – Metastasis in single regional lymph node, 2 cm or less in
      greatest dimension
N2 – Metastasis in single regional lymph node, more than 2 cm
      but not more than 5 cm in greatest dimension, or
N3 – Metastasis in regional lymph node more than 5 cm in
      greatest dimension.

Metastatic disease (M)

M0 – No distant metastases
M1 – Distant metastases
M1a – Non-regional lymph node(s)
M1b – Bone(s)
M1c – Other site(s).

Table 3.2 Gleason grading system

Grade	Histological characteristics	Probability of local progression over 10 years
Grades 1–4	Well-differentiated cancer	25%
Grades 5–7	Moderately differentiated cancer	50%
Grades 8–10	Poorly differentiated cancer	75%

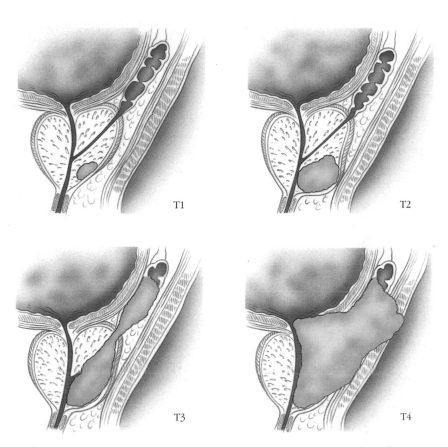

Figure 3.8 *Local staging of prostate cancer. The tumour may advance from T1 to T4 with or without the development of metastases.*

Grading prostate cancer

There are several systems of histological grading for prostate cancer, which are based on the degree of glandular differentiation, cytological atypia and nuclear abnormalities. The Gleason grading system (Table 3.2), which is the most widely used, provides one of the most clinically useful indicators of the likelihood of cancer progression, but is subject to variability of interpretation and sampling errors due to heterogeneity of tissue within the tumour.

The anatomical location of the cancer within the prostate may also be important; transition zone cancers may behave in a less aggressive fashion than those occurring in the peripheral zone.

Predicting the progression of early cancer

At present, those early prostate cancers that will progress to infiltrating carcinoma cannot be distinguished with absolute certainty from those that will remain occult within the patient's natural lifespan. Some insight into this dilemma has been gleaned from studying incidental cancers diagnosed at TURP. The median time to progression for T1a (low volume and well differentiated) and T1b (higher volume and moderately or poorly differentiated) carcinomas has been estimated at 13.5 and 4.75 years, respectively[15]. It has therefore become common practice to manage T1a disease in older men by 'watchful waiting' only. Men under 70 years, however, may well live long enough for clinical progression of the tumour to occur and therefore might be considered candidates for a more aggressive therapeutic approach. Much research endeavour is currently directed towards identifying molecular markers which will accurately predict prostate tumour progression and metastasis.

Pathology of prostatitis

Prostatitis is the third major source of prostatic pathology. It is characterized by inflammation of the prostate gland (Figure 3.9) and presents as both acute and chronic perineal pain. Prostatitis can be divided into four main syndromes:

- acute bacterial prostatitis
- chronic bacterial prostatitis
- chronic abacterial prostatitis
- prostatodynia.

Prostatitis usually occurs in the peripheral zone of the prostate, and is occasionally associated with necrosis and glandular atrophy and abscess formation.

Acute bacterial prostatitis is often caused by Gram-negative rods, such as *Escherichia coli* and *Pseudomonas aeruginosa,* and less commonly enterococci, such as *Streptococcus faecalis* (Gram-positive organisms).

Chronic bacterial prostatitis may be caused by a variety of organisms including *Escherichia coli, Klebsiella* spp., *Pseudomonas* spp.*, Mycoplasma hominis* and *Chlamydia trachomatis.* A history of preceding acute prostatitis is not always a feature.

The histological findings show less inflammatory reaction and more focal changes than in acute bacterial prostatitis, and there may be infiltration by plasma cells, macrophages and lymphocytes.

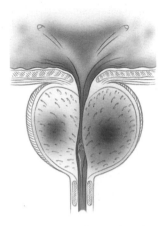

Figure 3.9 *Prostatitis. Bacterial or abacterial inflammation involves mainly the peripheral zone and may result in voiding symptoms and perineal pain.*

Chronic abacterial prostatitis. Many cases of chronic prostatitis are abacterial, in that no infecting organism can be demonstrated. This condition may be secondary to spasm, or increased pressure in the distal urethra or external sphincter. This pressure may lead to reflux of urine into the prostatic ducts, resulting in glandular and interstitial inflammation[16]. Once inflammation has occurred within the gland, it tends to become chronic with periods of remission and relapse.

Summary

■ BPH develops in the transitional zone of the prostate while both cancer and prostatitis usually develop in the peripheral zone.

■ After the age of 40, the appearance of microscopic stromal nodules marks the start of the development of BPH.

- In BPH, smooth muscle is a more common component of the stroma than glandular tissue; however, the balance of tissues affected varies from man to man, which may explain why prostate size is not related to severity of symptoms or obstruction.

- Serum PSA levels may be elevated in 25% of patients with BPH; unstable detrusor contractions may result in frequency, urgency and nocturia in 70% of obstructed patients.

- Prostatic enlargement due to BPH can ultimately lead to urinary retention and other serious pathologies.

- The Gleason histological grading system is a useful, though imperfect, predictor of the risks of cancer progression.

- Chronic prostatitis may be categorized as bacterial or abacterial, according to the findings on culture of the expressed prostatic secretions (EPS).

References

1 McNeal JE. Regional morphology and pathology of the prostate. *Am J Clin Pathol* 1968; **49**: 347–57.

2 Ball AJ, Feneley RCL, Abrams PH. The natural history of untreated 'prostatism'. *Br J Urol* 1981; **533**: 613–16.

3 Craigen AA, Hickling JB, Saunders CRG, Carpenter RG. Natural history of prostatic obstruction. A prospective survey. *J R Coll Gen Pract* 1969; **18**: 226–32.

4 Birkoff JD. Natural history of benign prostatic hypertrophy. In: Hinman F, Boyarsky S, eds. *Benign Prostatic Hypertrophy.* New York: Springer-Verlag, 1983: 5–12.

5 Drach GW, Layton TN, Binard WJ. Male peak urinary flow rate: relationship of volume voided and age. *J Urol* 1979; **122**: 210–14.

6 Gilpin SA, Gilpin CJ, Dixon JS, Gosling JA, Kirby RS. The effect of age on the autonomic innervation of the bladder. *Br J Urol* 1986; **58**: 378–81.

7 Bartsch G, Muller HR, Boerholzer M, Rohr HP. Light microscopic stereological analysis of the normal human prostate and benign prostatic hyperplasia. *J Urol* 1979; **122**: 487–91.

8 Stamey TA, Yang N, Hay AR, McNeal JE, Freiha FF, Redwine E. Prostate specific antigen as a serum marker for carcinoma of the prostate. *N Engl J Med* 1987; **317**: 909–16.

9   Abrams PH, Griffiths DJ. The assessment of prostatic obstruction from urodynamic measurements and from residual urine. *Br J Urol* 1979; **51**: 129–34.

10 Gilpin SA, Gosling JA, Barnard RJ. Morphological and morphometric studies of the human obstructed, trabeculated urinary bladder. *Br J Urol* 1985; **57**: 525–9.

11 Speakman MJ, Brading AF, Gilpin CJ, Dixon JS, Gilpin SA, Gosling JA. Bladder outflow obstruction: cause of denervation supersensitivity. *J Urol* 1987; **138**: 1461–7.

12 Department of Veterans Affairs cooperative study of transurethral resection for benign prostatic hyperplasia. A comparison of quality of life with patient reported symptoms and objective findings in men with benign prostatic hyperplasia. *J Urol* 1993; **150**: 1696–1700.

13 Malone PR, Cook A, Edmondson R, Gill MW, Shearer RJ. Prostatectomy: patients' perception and long-term follow-up. *Br J Urol* 1988; **61**: 234–8.

14 Wilson JMG, Kemp IW, Stein GW. Cancer of the prostate: do younger men have a poorer survival rate? *Br J Urol* 1984; **56**: 391–6.

15 Lowe BA, Listrom MB. Incidental carcinoma of the prostate: an analysis of the predictors of progression. *J Urol* 1988;**140**:1340–4.

16 Kirby RS, Lowe D, Bultitude MI, Shuttleworth KED. Intra-prostatic urinary reflux: an aetiological factor in abacterial prostatitis. *Br J Urol* 1982; **54**: 729–731.

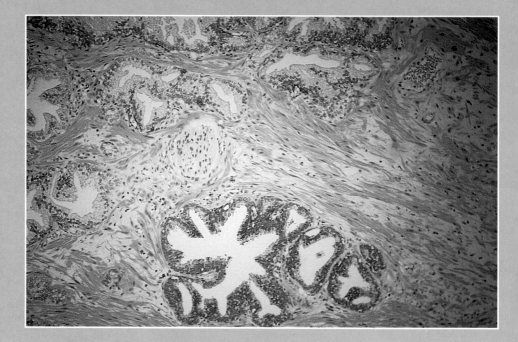

Chapter 4

Pathogenesis

Until the recent surge of interest in the pathogenesis of prostate diseases, only two factors had been shown to be absolute requirements for the development of benign prostatic hyperplasia (BPH):

■ androgen-producing normal testes

■ the influence of ageing.

It is now known, however, that a multiplicity of other factors are involved in the pathogenesis of BPH, although androgens clearly play a central role (Figure 4.1). The cascade of events which takes place from the stimulation of androgen secretion to the replication of cells is being elaborated, and it has been suggested that if a sufficient degree of disorganization of cellular control exists, these events may proceed to prostate cancer[1].

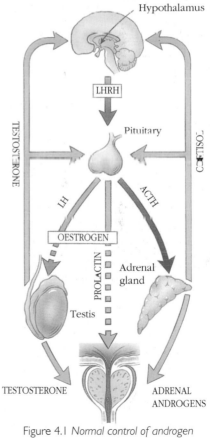

Figure 4.1 *Normal control of androgen production and utilization.*

BPH – the five theories

BPH is a disease that afflicts most ageing men; a number of theories for its pathogenesis have been suggested over recent years (Table 4.1).

Table 4.1 Theories for the cause of BPH

Theory	Cause	Effect
Dihydrotestosterone hypothesis	↑ 5-alpha reductase and androgen receptors	Epithelial and stromal hyperplasia
Oestrogen–testosterone imbalance	↑ Oestrogens ↓ Testosterone	Stromal hyperplasia
Stromal–epithelial interactions	↑ Epidermal growth factor/ fibroblast growth factor ↓ Transforming growth factor ß	Epithelial and stromal hyperplasia
Reduced cell death	↑ Oestrogens	↑ Longevity of stroma and epithelium
Stem cell theory	↑ Stem cells	Proliferation of transit cells

The dihydrotestosterone hypothesis

Dihydrotestosterone (DHT) is the principal intracellular androgen involved with the regulation of prostatic growth[2]. It is formed by the action of the enzyme 5-alpha reductase on testosterone within the prostate[3]. DHT is about five times more potent as an androgen within cells than testosterone, and it binds readily to the androgen receptors

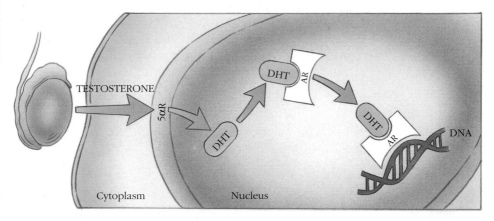

Figure 4.2 *The dihydrotestosterone (DHT) theory for the development of BPH. Testosterone produced by the testes enters the prostate cell and is metabolized by 5-alpha reductase (5αR) to DHT. This potent androgen then binds to androgen receptors (AR) and promotes cell growth.*

in the nucleus. This allows a sequence of events to take place within the cell which leads to cell replication (Figure 4.2).

Early studies suggested that tissue DHT levels were markedly increased in BPH compared to the normal prostate[4]. Although this would have provided an elegant explanation for the development of BPH, early hopes were dashed by further observations. The original studies had compared DHT levels in normal prostates with those in surgically removed BPH tissue. It was subsequently shown that these low levels in normal prostates resulted from autolysis, which could be reversed by incubating the tissue at body temperature for several hours, thus producing similar levels to those seen in surgically removed BPH tissue[5].

Increased 5-alpha-reductase activity. Although the level of DHT in BPH tissue is not elevated, it is very likely that 5-alpha-reductase activity and androgen receptor levels are greater in BPH tissue than in controls. It is the binding of DHT to the androgen receptors which is important in stimulating cell replication, and prostatic cells may therefore gradually become more sensitive to androgens with ageing, by virtue of the fact that the pathway to increased cell replication is accelerated.

Oestrogen–testosterone imbalance

The theory that an age-associated imbalance between circulating oestrogens and testosterone plays a role in the pathogenesis of BPH is attractive[6].

With ageing, the circulating level of free testosterone decreases gradually, while the level of free oestradiol remains unchanged. This results in a gradual, but significant, increase in the ratio of free oestradiol:free testosterone. It has been suggested that oestrogens may play a role in the genesis of BPH by sensitizing the prostate to androgens, either by causing an increase in the level of androgen receptors or by decreasing the rate of prostatic cell death. Oestrogens also cause hyperplasia of the stromal cells; oestrogens are produced principally by the aromatization of androgens. If the androgen drive to the prostate is ablated, 'apoptosis' (i.e. cell death) will occur and the prostate, especially its glandular elements, will involute and shrink.

Stromal–epithelial interactions

Interactions between the glandular and connective tissue elements of the prostate, stimulated by androgens, but effected by local growth factors, are an essential step in the pathogenesis of BPH.

The concept that a form of control of cell growth or inhibition can be influenced by the cell itself or by the surrounding tissues, is an essential part of the theory that prostatic stroma affects the growth of the prostatic epithelium. This effect of the stroma on the prostatic epithelial cells has been termed 'epithelial re-awakening'.

Experimental work has shown that the development of prostatic glandular tissue is indirectly controlled by androgens through mediators which arise from the stroma[7]. These are growth factors which are produced either by the prostatic epithelial cells or by the surrounding stroma. Examples include:

- epidermal growth factor (EGF)
- transforming growth factor alpha (TGF-alpha)
- fibroblast growth factor (FGF)
- TGF-beta (inhibitory).

Reduced cell death

A steady-state appears to exist after the prostate has reached its adult size, whereby the rates of prostatic cell growth and prostatic cell death are in equilibrium. This ensures that neither involution nor overgrowth takes place, so that prostate size is constant. The reduced cell death hypothesis suggests that the increased prostate volume in BPH is a function of a decrease in the rate of cell death perhaps in concert with an increase in cell proliferation (Figure 4.3). This hypothesis is also supported by the observation that BPH tissue has a lower than normal rate of mitotic activity.

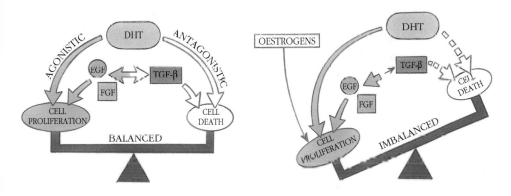

Figure 4.3 The reduced cell death theory proposes that BPH develops as a result of an imbalance of cell proliferation and cell death.

Stem cell theory

Stem cells. It is also possible that BPH results from abnormalities of cells within the prostate described as 'stem cells' (Figure 4.4). A stem cell is a proliferative cell, and the number of these cells within the prostate is unknown. The stem cells rarely divide, but on doing so produce an amplifying cell[8].

Amplifying cells proliferate and divide to only a limited degree, but these replications result in a major increase in the total number of cells present. Stem cells and amplifying cells are androgen independent, that is they do not require androgenic stimulation for their maintenance.

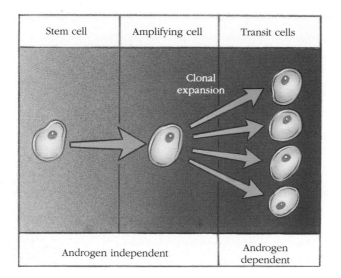

Stem cell	Amplifying cell	Transit cells

Clonal expansion

Androgen independent		Androgen dependent

Figure 4.4 *The stem cell theory for the development of BPH. Stem cells produce amplifying cells which, in turn, give rise to androgen-dependent transit cells.*

Transit cells. A third type of cell, the so-called transit cell is derived from the amplifying cells; they are capable of only limited proliferation, and this is determined by androgenic stimulation. The transit cells are the most common cells within the prostate and, because of their dependence on androgenic stimulation for proliferation and maintenance, they undergo apoptosis and disappear most quickly from the prostate after castration.

Completing the picture

The cause of BPH is complex, involving many steps, which are both intra- and extra-prostatic, and intra- and extracellular. Advances in our knowledge are taking place at an ever-increasing rate, and it is to be hoped that it will soon be possible to link together the various theories in order to complete the picture of the pathogenesis of BPH and elucidate its relationship to prostatic carcinoma.

Premalignant lesions of the prostate

Sometimes patients with ostensibly benign prostatic disease are followed-up on a regular basis by the urologist. One reason for this is

Figure 4.5 *Histological section of the prostate showing prostatic intra-epithelial neoplasia (PIN) within the glandular structure.*

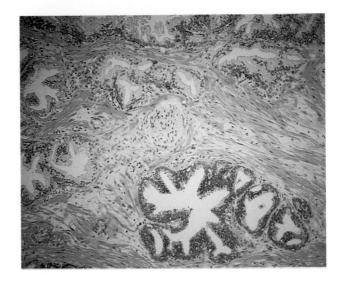

that the existence of premalignant lesions in the prostate may alert the urologist to the necessity that close follow-up rather than discharge back to family practitioners is required.

Prostatic intra-epithelial neoplasia

Prostatic intra-epithelial neoplasia (PIN) is associated with various alterations in prostatic cellular architecture which bridge the gap between a benign and malignant prostate (Figure 4.5). When these changes are present, they require careful follow-up as they are very likely to be a premalignant condition.

PIN consists of dysplastic foci present in the prostatic ducts and acini[9]. It occurs in about 40% of men who are over 50 years of age and who do not have a prostatic carcinoma, but rises to 80% in men who do have prostate cancer.

Prostate cancer

Although the exact cause of prostate cancer is unknown, recent discoveries link it inextricably to changes in the genetic structure of prostatic cells. Part of the problem in establishing the cause of prostatic carcinoma is the variability and heterogeneity of the tumour within the prostate gland. The following section gives a résumé of some of the work which has been performed to date.

Imbalance in growth regulation

As in BPH, stromal–epithelial interactions and growth factors may also play a role in the pathogenesis of malignant disease of the prostate. These important local regulatory factors are involved in a delicate balance which controls, not only cell growth, but also programmed cell death.

It is easy to see that the growth factors, which are produced not only by the target cells themselves, but also by cells located close to the target cells, could develop a significant imbalance which, if prolonged, would be an important step in the genesis of the cascade of events which ultimately leads to prostate cancer. In this way, it is conceivable that BPH itself is a premalignant condition, thus explaining the high incidence of microfoci of prostate cancer (which increases exponentially with time). As mentioned, this is as yet just an educated surmise, and does not mean that the many hundreds of thousands of patients with BPH should be followed-up routinely. It is nevertheless a fascinating area of future research.

Initiation of prostate cancer

It is clear that androgens provide the primary signal for DNA synthesis and cell division within the prostate. This is effected through a complex mechanism and is probably the case, not only in normal prostate, but also in BPH and prostate cancer. The signal is given through various growth factors which stimulate growth and differentiation of prostatic epithelial cells, and also in some cases act as a brake on further growth.

Proto-oncogene stimulation. The various growth factors are almost certainly involved in the stimulation of proto-oncogenes (Figure 4.6); these are normal cellular genes involved in the regulation of growth and cellular differentiation. This normal activity is also influenced by the surrounding tissues, and the neighbouring

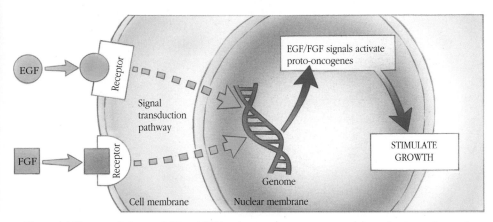

Figure 4.6 *The growth factors EGF and FGF activate proto-oncogenes and thus stimulate cell growth.*

normal cells exercise a restraint over the growth of abnormal cells within the prostate.

Carcinogenesis may develop when the genetic restraint and control in the growth of the cell is lost. This can happen, for example, when oncogenes develop as a result of changes in the normal proto-oncogenes. Abnormal intracellular behaviour can be induced by oncogene activation or by a change in activity or a change in character of the tumour suppressor genes. It is likely that malignant changes require abnormalities to coexist in more than one oncogene, for example *c ras* and *c myc*. The simultaneous activation of these oncogenes could override the inhibitory restraints of neighbouring cells and allow tumour proliferation.

Deletion of tumour suppressor genes. The normal cell contains genes which protect the individual against cancer, for example, *p53* and the *Rb* genes. It is known that loss of these genes may result in cancer, and it seems probable that the prostate tumours that occur in younger men, which appear to have a familial basis, may also be the result of specific gene deletions.

Cancer progression and androgen resistance

The concept that a normal prostate can progress through hyperplasia to malignancy can be taken somewhat further. For example, if normal growth regulation and control is imbalanced and hyperplasia develops, the introduction of genetic instability can lead to the initiation of prostate cancer, which can, in turn, proceed to local and metastatic progression. Many studies are under way to discover the conditions that are required for such progression to take place, and it would seem that many factors are involved.

Vascular development. The development of new capillary blood vessels (angiogenesis) might well be one of the first steps in cancer progression. This may be induced by the abnormal tumour expression of growth factors, for example, FGF.

Cadherins and cell adherence. Further progression and eventual metastasis may result from the fact that malignant cells are less adherent to one another than normal cells. Cadherins are cell surface glycoproteins that are required for cell adhesion. Changes in the gene which controls cadherins could well be involved in progression and metastasis[10].

Extension of the tumour into the extracellular matrix is probably a complex alteration involving integrins (mediators between the malignant cells and the adhesive proteins of the extracellular matrix), and fibronectin (which forms an important part of the basement membrane). If the malignant cell becomes attached through the mediation of integrin to the changed molecule of fibronectin, disease progression might occur.

Mitogenic cytokines are motility factors which are concerned with cell movement. If these motility factors (such as scatter factor and migration stimulating factor) deregulate the normal control of cellular migration, this might well account for the migration and metastasis of tumour cells. Although this is a very attractive hypothesis, the secretion of these motility factors from cancer cells has yet to be proven.

Genetic instability. In the growing tumour, the possibility of genetic instability is an important concept. This would allow the development of cell variants with different degrees of androgen sensitivity. Changes may take place which allow the development of androgen-insensitive cells and the death of androgen-sensitive cells.

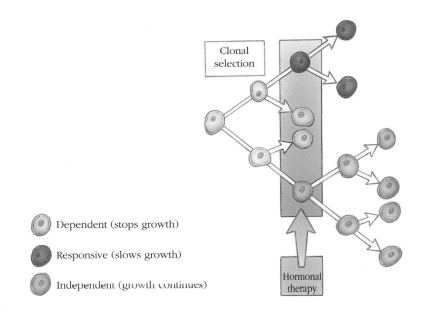

Figure 4.7 *Clonal selection: androgen-independent cells are selected out after hormonal therapy and grow to result in 'hormone escaped' prostate cancer.*

This would provide a further movement away from the modulating influence of androgens on the growth factors associated with normal cell regulation and the subsequent de-differentiation, not only of the cell type, but also of cellular activity (Figure 4.7).

Looking ahead

A flurry of activity is currently under way surrounding the mechanics of the regulation of prostate cell growth. These studies focus on the steady progression from normal control through local stimulation to various abnormalities in modulation of these processes and, ultimately, the development of BPH and cancer. Increased knowledge of the pathogenesis of prostatic disease in general will most likely lead to improved therapies in the future.

Summary

■ The aetiology of BPH is multifactorial and as yet not fully understood; ageing and the presence of androgens are definite requirements for its development.

■ The key androgen in the pathogenesis of BPH is DHT, which is produced by the action of 5-alpha reductase on testosterone within the prostatic cell.

■ BPH is likely to be related not only to increased activity of 5-alpha reductase and an increased number of androgen receptors within the prostatic cell nucleus, but also to an imbalance of free testosterone and free oestrogen in the blood.

■ Other views are that the rate of prostatic cell death and stromal–epithelial cell interactions are important in the pathogenesis of BPH. Oestrogens may play a role here.

■ The stem cell theory suggests BPH is caused by different types of cells within the prostate that proliferate at different rates due to different sensitivities to androgens.

■ Prostate cancer may arise from an imbalance in many growth factors affecting both stromal and epithelial growth.

■ Genetic causes of prostate cancer may involve changes to proto-oncogenes and tumour suppressor genes.

■ Vascular development, cellular adhesion molecules, motility factors and genetic changes causing androgen resistance may be involved in the progression of prostate cancer.

References

1   Griffiths K. Regulation of prostatic growth. In: Cockett ATK, Khoury S, Aso Y, Chatelain C, Denis L, Griffiths K, Murphy G, eds. *The 2nd international consultation on benign prostatic hyperplasia.* Paris: SCI, 1994: 49–75.

2   Bruchovsky N, Wilson JD. The conversion of testosterone to 5-alpha-androstan-17-beta-ol-3-one by rat prostate in vivo and in vitro. *J Biol Chem* 1968; **243**: 2012–21.

3   Anderson KM, Liao S. Selective retention of dihydrotestosterone by prostatic nuclei. *Nature* 1968; **219**: 277–9.

4   Siiteri PK, Wilson JD. Dihydrotestosterone metabolism in prostate hypertrophy. I. The formation of content of dihydrotestosterone in the hypertrophic prostate of man. *J Clin Invest* 1970; **49**: 1737–45.

5   Walsh PC, Hutchins GM, Ewing LL. Tissue content of dihydrotestosterone in human prostatic hyperplasia is not supranormal. *J Clin Invest* 1983; **72**: 1772–7.

6   Trachtenberg J, Hicks LL, Walsh PC. Androgen and estrogen receptor content in spontaneous and experimentally induced canine prostatic hyperplasia. *J Clin Invest* 1980; **65**: 1051–9.

7   Cunha R, Chung LWK, Shannon JM *et al.* Stromal-epithelial interactions in sex differentiation. *Biol Reprod* 1980; **22**: 19–42.

8   Isaacs JT. Control of cell proliferation and cell death in the normal and neoplastic prostate. A stem cell model. In: Roger CH, Coffey DS, Cuhna G *et al* eds. *Benign prostatic hyperplasia Vol 2* (NIH Publication 87–2881). US Department of Health and Human Services, Washington DC, 1987: 85–94.

9   Bostwick DG, Brawer MK. Prostatic intraepithelial neoplasia and early invasion in prostate cancer. *Cancer* 1987; **59**: 778–94.

10 Giroldi LA, Schalken JA. Decreased expression of the intercellular adhesion molecule E-cadherin in prostate cancer: biological significance and clinical implications. *Cancer and Metastasis Reviews* 1993, **12**. 29–37.

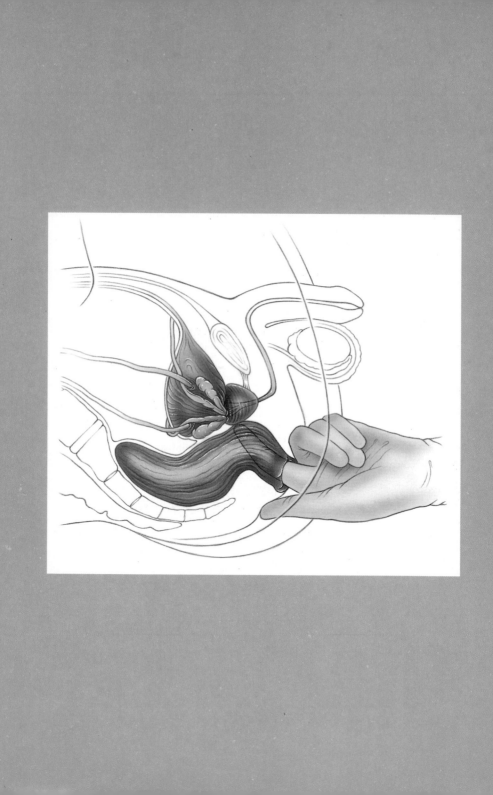

Chapter 5

Diagnosing prostatic disorders

Today, the diagnosis of prostatic disorders requires a methodical, multitechnical approach. Although not always perfect, these modern techniques provide useful information that helps to distinguish benign conditions from those more likely to be malignant. Some of these tests may also provide prognostic information about the likely natural history of the condition and the risk:benefit ratio of particular treatment options. It is worth bearing in mind the many risk factors for prostatic disease (Table 5.1) when making a diagnosis and, as always, the first step is to take a good history.

Table 5.1 Risk factors for clinical BPH and prostate cancer

BPH	Prostate cancer
■ Ageing	■ Age
■ Normal testicular function	■ Western life-style (? fats, red meat)
■ ? Increasing oestrogen levels	■ Afro-Caribbean extraction
■ ? Family history	■ First-degree relative(s) affected
■ ? Western diet/life-style	■ Age of first sexual intercourse
	■ Number of sexual partners
	■ Occupation (e.g. nuclear power workers)
	■ ? Vasectomy

History

Benign prostatic hyperplasia (BPH) is by far the most common diagnosis in men presenting with prostate problems. In practical terms, probably most cases of clinical BPH can be initially identified by asking three questions (Table 5.2). A family history of prostate cancer, especially in first-degree relatives, necessitates an especially thorough screening for prostate malignancy.

Table 5.2 The three questions for detecting prostatic disease

- Do you get up at night to pass urine?
- Is your urine flow slow?
- Are you bothered by your bladder function?

Classical symptoms

Both irritative and obstructive lower urinary tract symptoms (Table 5.3) are prevalent in ageing men and women. The symptom complex that characterizes symptomatic BPH is called 'prostatism'. Post-micturition dribble is a common symptom due to pooling of urine in the bulbar urethra and not closely associated with outflow obstruction.

Several structured symptom questionnaires have been developed to evaluate the severity of symptoms and their 'bothersomeness'. Points are assigned for each answer, the sum of which is the symptom score. Early examples of these scores were the Boyarsky[1] and the Madsen-Iversen[2] scores. However, these have now been superseded by the International Prostate Symptom Score (IPSS)[3] – which was originally developed by the American Urological Association (AUA) and recently adopted by the World Health Organization[4].

The International Prostate Symptom Score (IPSS) (Table 5.4) is simple and has been validated for test-retest reliability[5]. It can be completed by the patient either before seeing the doctor or during the consultation. However, correlation between other parameters of lower

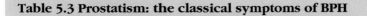

Table 5.3 Prostatism: the classical symptoms of BPH

Obstructive symptoms	Irritative symptoms
■ Hesitancy	■ Urgency
■ Weak stream*	■ Frequency
■ Straining	■ Nocturia
■ Prolonged micturition	■ Urge incontinence
■ Feeling of incomplete emptying*	
■ Urinary retention	
■ Overflow incontinence	

* Correlated most strongly with subsequent need for prostatectomy[6].

urinary tract dysfunction (e.g. flow rates and prostate volume) and symptom scores is not always good. Nevertheless, in patients proven to have bladder outflow obstruction due to BPH by other objective means, the IPSS does give a useful measure of both symptom severity and 'bothersomeness'. Specific symptoms that appear to correlate most strongly with the eventual need for prostatic surgery are poor flow and the sensation of incomplete emptying[6]

Chronic prostatitis typically occurs in younger men (35–50 years) who present with perineal ache, ejaculatory pain, dysuria and voiding dysfunction. Acute bacterial prostatitis causes symptoms typical of febrile illness, as well as those associated with prostatic disease .

Other important symptoms

Other urinary tract symptoms not included in the IPSS may also be important, though it should be remembered that localized, still curable, cancers of the prostate are usually asymptomatic.

Macroscopic haematuria indicates the need for referral for intravenous urography (IVU) and cystoscopy because of its strong association with malignant transitional cell carcinoma.

Table 5.4 International Prostate Symptom Score (IPSS)*

	Not at all	Less than 1 time in 5	Less than half the time	About half the time	More than half the time	Almost always	Patient score
1 Incomplete emptying Over the past month, how often have you had a sensation of not emptying your bladder completely after you finished urinating?	0	1	2	3	4	5	
2 Frequency Over the past month, how often have you had to urinate again less than 2 hours after you finished urinating?	0	1	2	3	4	5	
3 Intermittency Over the past month, how often have you found you stopped and started again several times when you urinated?	0	1	2	3	4	5	
4 Urgency Over the past month, how often have you found it difficult to postpone urination?	0	1	2	3	4	5	
5 Weak stream Over the past month, how often have you had a weak urinary stream?	0	1	2	3	4	5	
6 Straining Over the past month, how often have you had to push or strain to begin urination?	0	1	2	3	4	5	

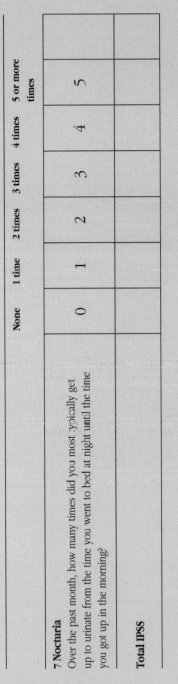

	None	1 time	2 times	3 times	4 times	5 or more times
7 Nocturia Over the past month, how many times did you most typically get up to urinate from the time you went to bed at night until the time you got up in the morning?	0	1	2	3	4	5
Total IPSS						

Interpretation of IPSS values

0–7 Mild; 8–18 Moderate; > 18 Severe. Total possible score = 35.

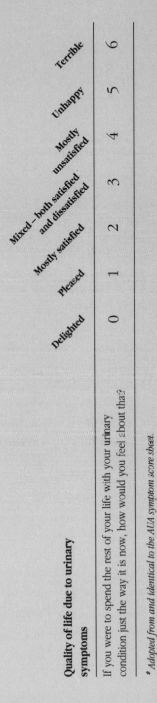

	Delighted	Pleased	Mostly satisfied	Mixed – both satisfied and dissatisfied	Mostly unsatisfied	Unhappy	Terrible
Quality of life due to urinary symptoms If you were to spend the rest of your life with your urinary condition just the way it is now, how would you feel about that?	0	1	2	3	4	5	6

* Adopted from and identical to the AUA symptom score sheet.

55

Dysuria or painful micturition may indicate urinary tract infection (UTI), but may also be the result of carcinoma *in situ* of the bladder. With the latter, urine cytology will often be positive for malignant cells.

Incontinence or enuresis in elderly men is often the result of chronic retention with overflow; however, a low-pressure, 'baggy' over-distended bladder may not always be easy to palpate.

Rapid onset of prostatism and low back pain suggest the presence of advanced prostate cancer, and necessitate immediate referral.

Physical examination

Abdomen

The abdomen should be examined in all patients with prostate problems to detect a palpable bladder.

Digital rectal examination

Digital rectal examination (DRE) provides the cornerstone of the physical assessment for prostate disease. It is the most simple and cost-effective method of assessing prostate health (Table 5.5), and has almost no morbidity.

DRE may be performed with the patient in the left lateral or knee-elbow position (Figure 5.1). The normal prostate is about the size of a chestnut and has the same rubbery consistency as the tip of the nose. BPH results in symmetrical enlargement with little alteration in consistency and preservation of the midline sulcus. By contrast, prostate cancer results in stony induration of the prostate that often starts as a palpable nodule and progresses to asymmetry of one lobe of the gland and eventually involvement and fixation of adjacent structures, especially the seminal vesicles which should normally be impalpable.

Rectal examination of a patient with acute prostatitis usually reveals a tender, sometimes 'boggy' prostate. The findings on DRE in patients with chronic bacterial prostatitis are variable, showing no abnormality, generalized tenderness or localized induration, which may be hard due to calcification or the presence of prostatic stones. The seminal vesicles and epididymes may also be indurated and tender.

As with any manual skill, accurate DRE of the prostate takes practice to acquire. The key to mastering the technique is to be gentle, take sufficient time and think about what you are doing. Even in expert hands, the positive predictive value of a palpable nodule turning out to be cancer on subsequent biopsy is only about 30%, but increases in direct proportion to the rise in serum prostate-specific antigen (PSA). It must be remembered, however, that it is quite possible for palpable cancer to be present when the PSA level is

Table 5.5 Clinical parameters that may be assessed by digital rectal examination

Size
Transverse and longitudinal dimension estimated, as well as posterior protrusion. The normal gland is the size of a chestnut (20 g). With BPH, the gland progressively enlarges to the size of a satsuma (> 50 g)

Consistency
Slight pressure applied smoothly while gliding over the surface of the gland to detect whether:
■ smooth or elastic - normal
■ hard or woody - may indicate cancer
■ tender - suggests prostatitis

Mobility
Attempts made to move the prostate up and down or to the sides. A malignant gland may be fixed to adjacent tissue

Anatomical limits
Finger used to try to reach lateral and cranial borders; medial sulcus carefully palpated. The seminal vesicles should be impalpable; induration of these suggests malignancy

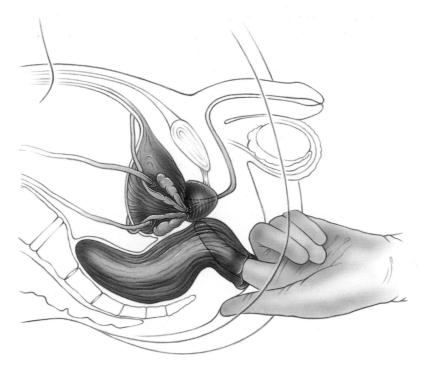

Figure 5.1 *Digital rectal examination (DRE) of the prostate should be performed in all patients presenting with prostate problems. Note that only the posterior portion of the gland is accessible to palpation.*

normal. Nevertheless, if the DRE is normal and the PSA less than 4.0 ng/ml, few patients will have clinically significant volumes of prostate cancer present. There is no evidence that DRE itself will cause a rise in serum PSA value.

Investigations

Urinalysis

Ideally, urinalysis should be performed in all men presenting with prostatism and, if positive, urine microscopy and culture carried out to exclude haematuria or urinary tract infection (UTI). Patients with particularly intractable irritative symptoms should also be considered for urine cytology to exclude transitional cell carcinoma.

Expressed prostatic secretions

The diagnosis of chronic prostatitis requires evidence of an excessive number of white (pus) cells in the expressed prostate secretions (EPS) following prostatic massage (Figure 5.2) or post-prostatic mass urine above that found in the first voided urine or in the midstream urine. A positive culture confirms bacterial rather than abacterial prostatitis. Patients with no objective evidence of an inflammatory condition are said to suffer from prostatodynia, the aetiology of which may be psychological.

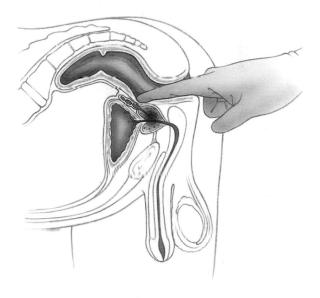

Figure 5.2 *Massaging the prostate. Prostatic secretions can be massaged into the urethra and collected for culture and sensitivity studies.*

Creatinine and electrolytes

Approximately 10% of patients with BPH seen by urologists have some degree of renal insufficiency. While the renal impairment is not always due to prostatic obstruction, it may influence the performance of other diagnostic tests, such as IVU and in itself suggests the need for more urgent treatment. It is therefore recommended that blood urea, electrolytes and creatinine values are determined as a safety check in all patients with prostatic symptoms.

Prostate-specific antigen (Table 5.6)

PSA is an imperfect serum marker for prostate cancer because it is so often mildly elevated in BPH. However, this test does identify a group of patients who are at risk of harbouring malignancy. While PSA testing is not mandatory in the evaluation of patients with prostatism, it is recommended in men under 75 years of age in whom the identification of prostate cancer would influence treatment decisions. There is no evidence that DRE increases the serum PSA level significantly and patients with prostatism may therefore have blood drawn for PSA estimation after this examination during their first visit.

Table 5.6 Features of prostate-specific antigen

- Glycoprotein whose function is to liquify semen
- Produced exclusively by prostatic epithelium
- Normal serum value < 4.0 ng/ml
- Elevated in 25% of patients with BPH
- Increased in most cases of prostate cancer
- Tends to rise progressively with age and prostatic volume

Interpreting PSA (Table 5.7). If the PSA value is greater than 10 ng/ml, then the chance of the patient having cancer on biopsy is about 60%[7]; however, only about 2% of patients with BPH have PSA values above 10 ng/ml. By contrast, if the PSA is between 4.1 and 10 ng/ml, then the risk of cancer on prostatic biopsy falls to around 20%[8]. This is because minor PSA elevations in the 4–10 ng/ml range are present in about 25% of patients with histologically proven BPH, and about 70–80% of patients with localized, significant volume prostate cancer[9]. Overall then, if the PSA is greater than 4 ng/ml, the likelihood of prostate cancer is in the region of 25–30%.

Patients with a raised PSA and/or abnormal DRE findings should therefore be referred for further study and biopsy unless they are so

Table 5.7 Interpretation of prostate-specific antigen (PSA) values

PSA value	Interpretation
0.5–4 ng/ml	Normal
4–10 ng/ml	20% chance of cancer
> 10 ng/ml	50%+ chance of cancer
Rise of > 20%/year	Refer immediately for biopsy

old, or otherwise unwell, that treatment of any cancer detected may not be indicated. It should be remembered that BPH is at least 10 times more prevalent than significant volume adenocarcinoma of the prostate. Recent data have, however, demonstrated the inability of a single estimation of PSA to clearly separate men with organ-confined cancer from those with BPH[10]. A number of strategies have therefore been evolved to enhance the accuracy of the PSA test as an indicator of cancer.

PSA density. Calculation of a PSA density (PSAD) depends on the observation that the PSA values in BPH tend to rise proportionately to the volume of the gland. Thus, a correction for the BPH contribution to the PSA value can be made by dividing the PSA value by the gland volume (in cm^3), as calculated by transrectal ultrasound (TRUS), to give the PSAD[11]. Values above 0.15 are regarded as suspicious of malignancy.

This concept is criticized on the grounds that not all BPH tissues elaborate predictable quantities of PSA, and that TRUS measurements of prostate volume are operator dependent and themselves subject to significant variability.

The PSA slope is formed by measuring and plotting sequential PSA values (Figure 5.3). As 'clinically significant' prostate cancer is composed of actively dividing cells which elaborate PSA, while normal prostate and BPH have only very slow cell division rates, patients with prostate cancer might be expected to show sequential PSA rises.

This was confirmed in a small retrospective study[12], which showed that men with normal prostates or BPH had stable PSA values, while

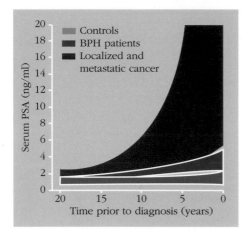

Figure 5.3 *Comparison of increases in serum PSA levels with time prior to the diagnosis of the prostate condition.*

those with carcinoma showed progressive rises. It was suggested that a rise of more than 20% or an increase of 0.75 ng/ml over 1 year was indicative of prostate cancer. In addition, in a screening follow-up study, the technique seemed to enhance the diagnostic yield[13]. However, as the interassay estimation of PSA values is subject to a variation of 8–15% in the same patient[14], more than two individual values may be necessary to obtain a true picture of the PSA slope.

Age-adjusted PSA cut-off values. Serum PSA values tend to increase very gradually with age[15]. This is probably the result of slowly developing BPH, but could also be due to more PSA 'leaking' from prostatic gland lumina into the plasma as the normal cell barriers break down with time. A line drawn through the 95th percentile for PSA values in a population in which prostate cancer had been excluded produced the age-adjusted cut-offs shown in Table 5.8. It has been argued that these cut-off values could serve to increase diagnostic

Table 5.8 Recommended age-adjusted prostate-specific antigen (PSA) cut-off values

Age (years)	PSA cut-off value (ng/ml)
40-49	2.5
50-59	3.5
60-69	4.5
70-79	6.5

suspicion in younger men in whom a diagnosis of prostate cancer may be more important, because of their longer life expectancy. While such a manoeuvre may improve the sensitivity of PSA testing, it probably does so at the price of reduced specificity. This raises the possibility of leaving some cancers undiagnosed, but this, especially in older age groups, may be desirable.

More cancer-specific PSA tests. PSA is a powerful protease which, when present in plasma in a concentration of 1 million times less than in seminal fluid, is largely bound to one of two inhibitors:

- alpha-1 antichymotrypsin
- alpha-2 macroglobulin.

Alpha-2 macroglobulin completely envelopes the PSA molecule and shields all the antigen from the antibody assay, while the alpha-1 antichymotrypsin shields only some of the antigenic surfaces (Figure 5.4), thus enabling the various bound and unbound forms to be distinguished.

It has recently been reported that differential amounts of the conjugated versus unconjugated PSA are present in patients with prostate cancer compared with those with BPH[16, 17]. This observation raises the prospect of a more cancer-specific PSA assay in the near future.

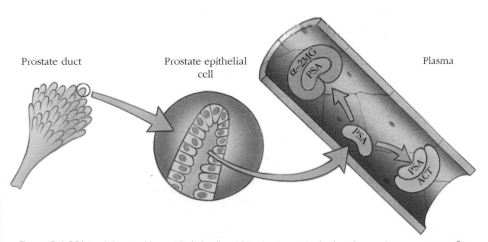

Prostate duct   Prostate epithelial cell   Plasma

Figure 5.4 *PSA is elaborated by epithelial cells within the prostate. In the plasma, it may occur as free PSA or conjugated to either alpha-1 antichymotrypsin (ACT) or alpha-2 macroglobulin (α-2MG).*

In considering the value of PSA testing, it is necessary to judge the ability of the test to distinguish those men who have only BPH from those who also have prostate cancer. In this respect, a single measurement of serum PSA is often inconclusive.

Uroflow measurement

The measurement of urinary flow rates using a flowmeter is simple, inexpensive, non-invasive and reasonably reproducible. The patient is asked to pass urine into a funnel and a printout is obtained. Although most family practices are not currently equipped with flowmeters, there is no reason why they should not be in the future. Modern flowmeters are unobtrusive and produce not only a flow trace, but also a computerized read-out listing the key parameters (Figure 5.5). It is, however, important that the voided volume exceeds

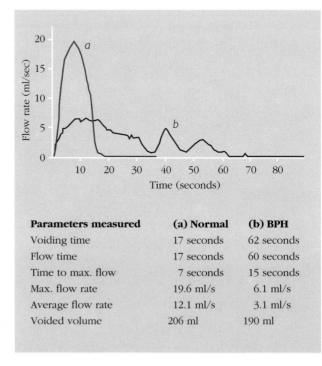

Parameters measured	(a) Normal	(b) BPH
Voiding time	17 seconds	62 seconds
Flow time	17 seconds	60 seconds
Time to max. flow	7 seconds	15 seconds
Max. flow rate	19.6 ml/s	6.1 ml/s
Average flow rate	12.1 ml/s	3.1 ml/s
Voided volume	206 ml	190 ml

Figure 5.5 (a) Normal flow rate tracing. (b) Flow rate tracing showing a reduction in the maximum flow rate in a patient with bladder outflow obstruction due to BPH.

150 ml – a requirement that may not always be easy to achieve in a patient with BPH with urinary frequency and a large post-void residual (PVR) volume. Small voided volumes may give erroneously low flow values. Also, an overfilled bladder may cause abnormal flow readings, especially in patients with severe obstruction.

Maximum flow rate, expressed in ml/second, is the most important variable in assessing obstruction. A measurement below the cut-off value of 15 ml/second suggests obstruction, and, in a younger man, a value below 10 ml/second is almost diagnostic (Table 5.9).

Table 5.9 Interpretation of maximum urinary flow rate values

Flow rate	Interpretation
> 15 ml/second	Normal
10–15 ml/second	Equivocal
< 10 ml/second	Obstructed

Maximum and mean urinary flow rates decrease gradually with age and a maximum flow of between 10 and 15 ml/second may be 'normal' in men 70–80 years of age[18]. In general, the lower the maximum flow rate, especially in younger men, the higher the probability of bladder outlet obstruction, which is predominantly caused by BPH. It must be remembered that the flow rate produced externally is a reflection of not only the outflow resistance, but also the power of detrusor contraction. Reduced detrusor contractility therefore, such as occurs in diabetes mellitus due to autonomic neuropathy and also with ageing, may result in a low uroflow. Conversely, an over-pronounced detrusor response to obstruction may produce a so-called 'high pressure–high flow' scenario – only urodynamics can elucidate these unusual entities.

Measurement of residual urine

As with a sub-optimal urine flow rate, an increased post-void residual (PVR) volume, which is best measured non-invasively by transabdominal ultrasound, may result from either infravesical obstruction or reduced detrusor contractility. Although informative, PVR values vary considerably from day to day and even from void to void[19]. The explanation for this is not clear, and therefore treatment decisions should not be made on the basis of this test alone. While the test cannot be used to confirm or refute a diagnosis of BPH, it is a useful safety parameter. The fact that patients with large PVR volumes are more likely to develop urinary retention makes them candidates for active treatment interventions rather than watchful waiting. PVR values consistently greater than 200–300 ml usually indicate the need for surgical rather than medical therapy.

Pressure/flow urodynamics

Pressure/flow urodynamics provide the only certain way of distinguishing outflow obstruction from failing detrusor contractility; however, the extent to which they should be used to confirm bladder outflow obstruction in BPH is controversial. While flow rate measurement is straightforward, recording of detrusor pressure during filling and voiding requires either urethral or suprapubic catheterization, which many patients dislike. The key parameter of obstruction is the detrusor pressure at maximum flow (i.e. the pressure within the bladder generated by the contracting bladder muscle minus rectal pressure to correct for artefact resulting from abdominal straining). Knowledge of both detrusor pressure and maximum flow rate allows the Abrams/Griffiths nomogram to be used to classify the patient as obstructed, unobstructed or equivocal.

Urodynamics are, however, time-consuming and expensive, and current consensus suggests these invasive tests should be confined to:

- patients with equivocal findings in whom surgery to relieve the outflow obstruction is seriously contemplated
- patients in placebo-controlled, randomized trials of new therapeutic modalities for prostatic obstruction.

Transrectal ultrasound of the prostate

TRUS has two potential values in evaluating patients with prostatism.

■ It permits reasonably accurate measurement of both the total gland and the transition zone volume.

■ It may reveal hypo-echoic foci in the peripheral zone suggestive of prostate cancer (Figure 5.6).

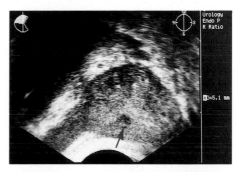

On biopsy, however, many of these hypo-echoic foci prove to be non-malignant, and conversely many cancers are iso-echoic or hyper-echoic. Because of its limited sensitivity and specificity, TRUS is not suitable as a first-line screening test for prostate cancer[20].

Figure 5.6 *Transrectal ultrasound scan showing a hypo-echoic focal lesion which proved on biopsy to be a carcinoma of the prostate.*

Prostatic biopsy. When DRE and/or PSA abnormalities are present, TRUS provides the most convenient and accurate way of

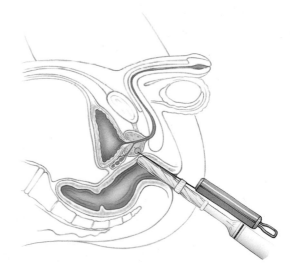

Figure 5.7 *Transrectal ultrasound (TRUS)-guided prostatic biopsy using an automated biopsy gun.*

obtaining prostatic biopsies. An automatic biopsy needle is advanced transrectally under ultrasound control and sextant prostate biopsies are taken (Figure 5.7). With adequate antibiotic cover, the morbidity of transrectal biopsy is minimal, though septic complications may occur in 2% of patients[21].

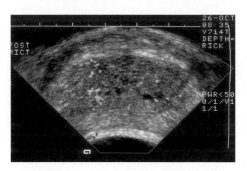

Figure 5.8 *Colour Doppler image showing diffuse hypervascularity in the peripheral zone of the prostate due to chronic prostatitis.*
(Courtesy of Dr David Rickards, Middlesex Hospital, London, UK.)

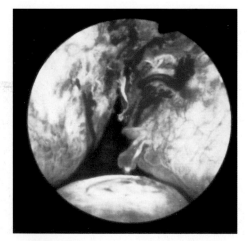

Figure 5.9 *Endoscopic view of lower urinary tract showing the lateral lobes of the prostate in a patient with BPH.*

Colour Doppler imaging can demonstrate blood flow through tissues, and therefore visualize inflammatory conditions of the prostate, such as acute and chronic prostatitis (Figure 5.8) and prostatic abscesses. In some cases, neovascularization in prostatic neoplasms may also be apparent and this technology may assist selection of areas to biopsy.

Endoscopy of the lower urinary tract

Endoscopy is not indicated in simple cases of clinical BPH, but does provide information about prostatic proportions (Figure 5.9). This information can, however, be obtained by TRUS, and cystoscopy should be confined to the investigation of patients in whom concomitant pathology, such as transitional cell carcinoma of the bladder is suspected, not least because the passage of a cystoscope in an obstructed patient may itself induce haematuria or even urinary retention.

Imaging of the upper urinary tracts

Imaging of the upper urinary tracts by IVU or ultrasonography is not routinely indicated in clinical BPH, because the diagnostic yield is so low. It is, however, appropriate in patients with:

- haematuria (either microscopic or macroscopic)
- recurrent UTIs
- renal, ureteric or bladder stones
- renal insufficiency.

Staging prostate cancer

Biopsy

As in other areas of cancer management, biopsy is essential to confirm the presence of malignant disease. The tissue cores usually provide sufficient material for the pathologist to give some indication of the degree of tumour differentiation, though not always enough for the calculation of a formal Gleason score (see page 30).

Prostate-specific antigen and transrectal ultrasound

PSA values above 50 ng/ml are usually but not invariably associated with metastases. TRUS results may be informative, but scans providing more anatomical detail are required to establish whether the tumour is still confined to the prostate, or whether bone or soft tissue metastases have already occurred.

Magnetic resonance imaging

The latest MRI technology with endorectal coils produces exquisite images of the prostate and can clearly demonstrate capsular involvement as well as seminal vesicle infiltration (Figure 5.10). MRI scanning can also reveal internal iliac node involvement by a tumour. Unfortunately, MRI scanning is

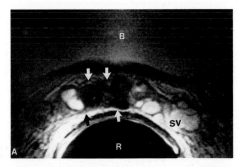

Figure 5.10 *Magnetic resonance imaging of the prostate showing seminal vesicle (SV) invasion. (B-bladder; R-rectum.)*

time-consuming and expensive. Furthermore, not all patients can tolerate the claustrophobic atmosphere within the scanner, and those with pacemakers, hip replacements or other metal-containing implants cannot be scanned.

CT scanning

CT scans can also demonstrate internal iliac node enlargement, and have the advantage over MRI of permitting skinny-needle aspiration to confirm malignant involvement. Obviously, microscopic nodal involvement cannot be detected. In practice, this is considered only when treatment decisions, such as whether or not to proceed to radical retropubic prostatectomy, hinge on the result.

Bone scanning

Bone scans (see page 152) are an important part of staging prostate cancers; however, they are rarely positive if the PSA is below 20 ng/ml and almost never when it is less than 10 ng/ml. Most urologists still routinely employ this test at the time of diagnosis for definitive confirmation or exclusion of skeletal deposits.

Guidelines for diagnosing prostatic disease

In an increasingly cost-conscious healthcare environment, it is important to avoid uninformative and unnecessary investigations. Although tests must always be chosen specifically for the patient concerned, general guidelines can be given for diagnosing prostatic disease[22,23].

Diagnosing benign prostatic hyperplasia (Figure 5.11)

Patients presenting with prostatism, identified by case finding or using the 'three questions' or who are seeking reassurance about their prostate, should be asked to complete a symptom score sheet (e.g. IPSS), as well as undergo a detailed history and examination, including a DRE. Urine should be analysed using the dipstick method and, if positive, an MSU obtained. Blood should be taken for urea,

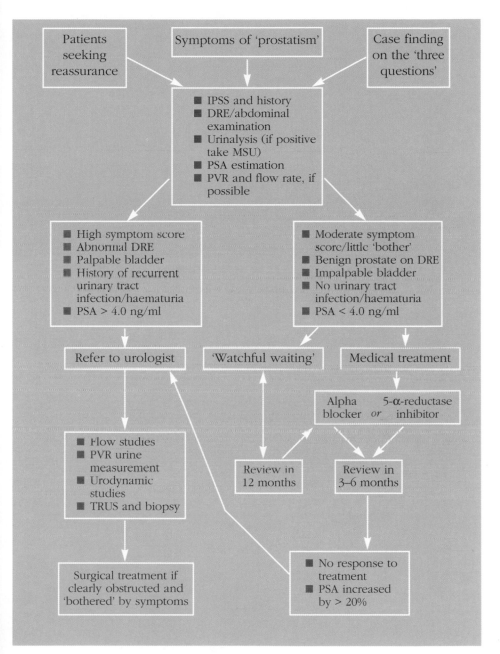

Figure 5.11 *Guidelines for diagnosing BPH.*

electrolytes and creatinine estimation; a PSA determination is optional but recommended in men under 75 years of age. The following findings suggest the need for the family practitioner to refer the patient urgently to a urologist:

■ IPSS > 18
■ history of haematuria or UTIs
■ suspicious-feeling prostate or a palpable bladder
■ PSA > 4.0 ng/ml.

Diagnosing prostate cancer (Figure 5.12)

Most patients suspected of harbouring prostate cancer are identified by either a suspicious DRE or a raised PSA. In either (or both) circumstance(s), the patient should be referred urgently for specialist evaluation including TRUS and usually biopsy. If the biopsy is negative, surveillance is all that is required. If the biopsy confirms adenocarcinoma, and provided active treatment would be indicated when the patient's age and life expectancy are accounted for, then staging investigations, including a bone scan or CT/MRI scans should be considered.

Diagnosing prostatitis (Figure 5.13)

Symptoms of perineal ache and pain on ejaculation should prompt the family practitioner to consider a diagnosis of prostatitis. DRE may reveal localized prostatic tenderness. The key to accurate diagnosis is the expression of EPS obtained by prostatic massage. A positive culture confirms bacterial prostatitis, the presence of white blood cells (WBCs) only suggests abacterial prostatic inflammation. The absence of either a positive culture or WBCs suggests 'prostatodynia' – or unexplained prostatic pain syndrome. Acute prostatitis may be associated with a transient rise in PSA; appropriate treatment should normalize PSA values within 6–12 weeks. Specialist referral for colour Doppler TRUS examination and biopsy should be considered if there is no response to therapy or PSA values remain above 4 ng/ml.

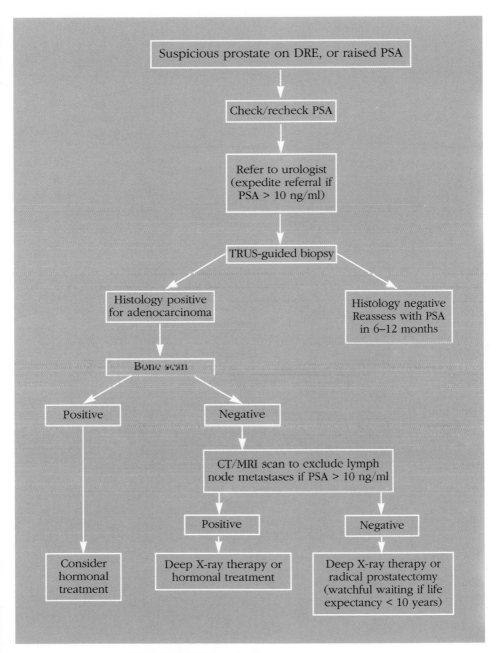

Figure 5.12 *Guidelines for diagnosing prostate cancer.*

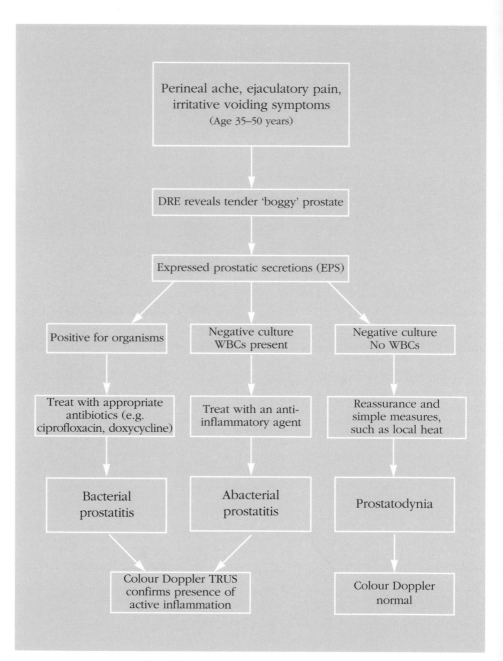

Figure 5.13 *Guidelines for diagnosing prostatitis.*

Summary

	BPH	**Prostate cancer**	**Prostatitis**
Symptoms	'Prostatism'	Asymptomatic until advanced	Dysuria Perineal ache Pain on ejaculation
DRE	Rubbery generalized enlargement	Stony hard induration	Tender 'boggy' prostate
PSA	Normal (75%) 4–10 ng/ml (25%) > 10 ng/ml (2%)	> 4 ng/ml (> 80%)	Sometimes ↑ Normalizes after antibiotics
Uroflow	↓	–	Sometimes ± ↓
PVR	↑	Sometimes ↑	Absent
EPS	Negative	Negative	Positive for organisms or WBCs
Urodynamics	↑ Voiding pressure ↓ Uroflow	– –	– –
TRUS/biopsy	BPH	Adenocarcinoma	Inflammation
Bone scan	–	Positive if bony metastases present	–
CT/MRI	–	Positive if large-volume lymph node metastases present	–

References

1 Boyarsky S, Jones G, Paulson DF, Front CR. A new look at bladder neck obstruction by the Food and Drug Administration regulators: Guidelines for investigation of benign prostatic hypertrophy. *Trans American Association of Genito-Urinary Surgeons* 1977; **68**: 29–32.

2 Madsen PO, Iversen PA. A point system for selecting operative candidates. In: Hinman FJr, Boyarsky S, eds. *Benign Prostatic Hypertrophy*. New York: Springer-Verlag, 1983; 763–9.

3 Barry MJ, Fowler FJ, O'Leary MP *et al*. The American Urological Association symptom index for benign prostatic hyperplasia. *J Urol* 1992; **148**: 1549–57.

4 Cockett ATK, Khoury S, Aso Y, Chatelain C, Denis L, Griffiths K, Murphy G, eds. *The 2nd international consultation on benign prostatic hyperplasia*. Paris: SCI, 1994.

5 Barry MJ, Fowler FJ, O'Leary MP, Bruskewitz RC, Holtgrewe HL, Mebust WK. Correlation of the American Urological Association symptom index with self-administered versions of the Madsen-Iversen, Boyarsky, and Maine Medical Assessment Program symptom indexes. *J Urol* 1992; **148**: 1558–63.

6 Arrighi HM, Guess HA, Metter EJ, Fozard JL. Symptoms and signs of prostatism as risk factors for prostatectomy. *Prostate* 1990; **16**: 253–61.

7 Catalona WJ, Smith DS, Ratliff TL *et al*. Measurement of prostate specific antigen in serum as a screening test for prostate cancer. *N Eng J Med* 1991; **324(17)**: 1156–61.

8 Oesterling JE. Prostate-specific antigen: improving its ability to diagnose early prostate cancer. *JAMA* 1992; **267**: 2236–8.

9 Oesterling JE. Prostate specific antigen: a critical assessment of the most useful tumour marker for adenocarcinoma of the prostate. *J Urol* 1991; **145**: 907–23.

10 Sherson P, Barry MJ, Oesterling JE. Serum PSA values in men with histologically confirmed BPH versus patients with localised prostate cancer. *J Urol* 1993; **149**: 412A.

11 Benson MC, Whang IS, Panteuck A *et al*. Prostate specific antigen density; a means of distinguishing between benign prostatic hypertrophy and prostate cancer. *J Urol* 1992; **147**: 815–16.

12 Carter HB, Pearson JD, Metter J *et al*. Longitudinal evaluation of prostate specific antigen levels in men with and without prostate cancer. *JAMA* 1993; **267**: 2215–20.

13 Brawer MK, Beatie J, Wener MH, Vessela RL, Preston SD, Lange PH. Screening for prostatic carcinoma with prostate specific antigen: results of the second year. *J Urol* 1993; **150**: 106–9.

14 Guess HA, Heyse JF, Gormley GJ. The effect of finasteride on prostate specific antigen in men with benign prostatic hyperplasia. *Prostate* 1993; **22**: 31–7.

15 Oesterling JE, Jacobsen SJ, Chute CG *et al*. Serum prostate-specific antigen in a community-based population of healthy men. *JAMA* 1993; **270**: 860–4.

16 Christensson A, Bjork T, Nilsson. Serum prostate specific antigen complexed to alpha-1 antichymotrypsin as an indicator of prostatic cancer. *J Urol* 1993; **150**: 100–5.

17 Bjartell A, Abrahamsson PA, Bjork T, Sant'Agnese A, Matikainen MT, Lilja H.

Production of alpha-1 antichymotrypsin by PSA-containing cells of prostate epithelium. *Urology* 1993; **43**: 502–10.

18 Girman CJ, Panser LA, Chute CG *et al.* Natural history of prostatism:urinary flow rates in a community based study. *J Urol* 1993; **150**: 887–92.

19 Bruskewitz RC, Iversen P, Madsen PO. Value of postvoid residual urine determination in evaluation of prostatism. *Urology* 1982; **20**: 602–4.

20 Terris MK, Freiha FS, McNeal JE, Stamey TA. Efficacy of transrectal ultrasound for identification of clinically undetected prostate cancer. *J Urol* 1991; **146**: 78–84.

21 Desmond PM, Clark V, Thompson IM, Zeidman EJ, Mueller EJ. Morbidity with contemporary prostate biopsy. *J Urol* 1993; **150**: 1425–6.

22 McConnell J *et al.* Benign prostatic hyperplasia: diagnosis and treatment. Agency for Health Care Policy and Research, Rockville MA, USA, 1994.

23 Roehrborn CG, Kurth KH, Leriche A *et al.* Diagnostic recommendations for clinical practice. In: Cockett ATK, Khoury S, Aso Y *et al.* eds. *The 2nd international consultation on benign prostatic hyperplasia,* Paris: SCI, 1993, 269–343.

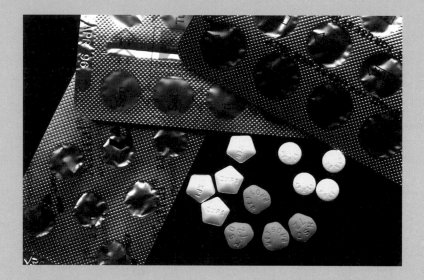

Chapter 6

Medical management of BPH

Shared care is now an increasingly important concept in the management of benign prostatic hyperplasia (BPH) for a number of reasons, including the increasing prevalence of the disease and the introduction of several pharmacological agents that have been shown to offer a safe and effective treatment option for many patients. For shared care to be successful, closer links between the primary care physician and the urologist are paramount.

Although transurethral resection of the prostate (TURP) is still the established treatment for patients with symptomatic BPH, alternative treatments should be considered for at least some patients for a number of reasons.

■ Firstly, postoperative morbidity appears, superficially, to be rather higher than expected, with an overall complication rate of about 15–16%[1]. In one study, long-term mortality after TURP also appeared to be higher than expected, but this may have been because co-morbidity was not satisfactorily excluded.

■ Secondly, 10–20% of patients who undergo TURP for BPH require a second procedure within 10 years, either to re-treat the condition, or to treat complications[2].

■ The third possible criticism of the acceptance of TURP as the standard treatment for all patients with symptomatic BPH is based on the observation that the prevalence of the disease is much higher than had been suspected[3]. It appears that the number of symptomatic men presenting to the urologist is only the tip of the iceberg, and that, if a less invasive method of treatment were available, many more men would perhaps come forward.

■ Fourthly, there appears to be considerable variation in the prostatectomy rate from country to country and even within individual countries[4]. In some locations, too many prostatectomies may, therefore, be being performed.

Approach to management

Treatment decisions for patients with symptomatic BPH should ideally be made by:

■ considering the nature and severity of the symptoms

■ assessing the 'bothersomeness' of symptoms and their impact on quality of life

■ determining whether urinary flow is significantly lowered and associated with a significant volume of post-void residual (PVR) urine.

Medical therapy is now a legitimate first-line treatment with acceptable results. Indeed, the symptomatic improvement achieved by medical treatment is often comparable to that of TURP, though it should be noted that improvement in peak flow rates is nearly always better after surgical treatment. Medical therapy is, however contraindicated in patients with certain specific pathologies (Table 6.1)

Medical treatment (Table 6.2) is probably most appropriate for patients with mild-to-moderate symptoms of BPH and, in our opinion, should be used as a specific treatment, rather than as an interim

---

Table 6.1 Contraindications for medical treatment of BPH

■ Urinary retention – acute or chronic
■ Renal insufficiency/upper tract dilatation
■ Recurrent haematuria
■ Recurrent urinary tract infections (UTIs) secondary to BPH
■ Bladder stones/diverticula

Table 6.2 Medical therapies for BPH (effects confirmed in placebo-controlled trials)

	Agent	Dose	Onset of action	Mechanism of action	Adverse effects
5-alpha-reductase inhibitors	Finasteride	5 mg/day	3–6 months	↓ Prostate volume	Impotence (3–5%)
	Epristeride	80 mg/day	3–6 months	Reverse BPH	
Alpha-1 blockers	Prazosin*	2 mg/day b.d.			Drowsiness and headache (10–15%)
	Doxazosin**	4 mg/day			
	Alfuzosin*	7.5 mg/day	2–4 weeks	Relax prostatic smooth muscle	Dizziness
	Terazosin**	5 mg/day			Postural hypotension (2–5%)
	Tamsulosin**	0.4 mg/day			

*Shorter acting.
**Longer acting.

measure while waiting for TURP. Currently, the main possibilities for the medical treatment of BPH are:

- alpha blockers
- androgen suppression.

Phytotherapy is also used in the management of BPH on an empirical, rather than a scientific basis, in many countries.

5-alpha-reductase inhibitors and alpha blockers have been thoroughly evaluated for safety and efficacy, and certainly have a role to play in the management of mild-to-moderately symptomatic BPH. It is strongly recommended that, before starting on this form of treatment, the following tests are carried out:

- International Prostate Symptom Score (IPSS)
- digital rectal examination (DRE)
- prostate-specific antigen (PSA)
- creatinine
- urinary flow rate.

Both types of therapeutic agent will improve symptom score and peak flow rate, and their effect may in theory be synergic. The value of combination therapy with both these classes of drugs is currently being tested in two major studies of terazosin/finasteride and doxazosin/finasteride.

Follow-up

Patients who are prescribed medical therapy for BPH should be carefully followed-up and reassessed on a regular basis, in order to ensure that their improvement is maintained, and that no other form of intervention is required. Symptomatic evaluation and peak flow rates should be performed every 6 months. PSA levels should be assessed every 6–12 months, especially in patients receiving finasteride which causes a mean reduction in PSA of 50% in patients with BPH, but a lesser decline or rise in those with prostate cancer.

Alpha blockers

The use of alpha blockers in the treatment of BPH has been invest-igated in a number of randomized placebo-controlled multicentre studies, which have demonstrated an early onset of action and lasting improvement in both symptoms and flow rates. Alpha blockers are a legitimate and satisfactory method of treating symptomatic BPH, with a relatively low incidence of side-effects (Table 6.3). Symptomatic improvement should be seen within the first 2–3 weeks of treatment and, if not seen within 3–4 months despite adequate dose titration, alternative therapy should be considered. If the patient is found to have significant symptomatic improvement, some reduction in PVR urine and an improvement in peak urinary flow, and the side-effects are not troublesome, treatment with these agents may be continued indefinitely.

Table 6.3 Effects of alpha blockers

- Usually require gradual dose titration
- Improve most symptoms of prostatism
- Enhance uroflow by 3–5 ml/sec
- Effective in around 60% of patients
- Produce drowsiness and headaches in 10–15% of patients
- Result in postural hypotension in 2–5% of patients

Mode of action

Contrary to what might be expected, BPH tissue consists, to a large degree, of an increase in both connective tissue and smooth muscle which is richly endowed with alpha receptors (Figure 6.1)[5]. This fact makes it easier to understand how norepinephrine (noradrenaline) can cause contraction of both the prostatic adenoma and of the capsule itself. There is, therefore, a clear rationale for the use of alpha blockade in the treatment of the dynamic component of bladder outflow obstruction; alpha blockers should improve outflow obstruction by decreasing outflow resistance without interfering with detrusor contractility. The newer alpha blockers have improved side-effect profiles and are also longer acting.

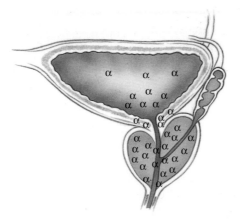

Figure 6.1 *Distribution of alpha receptors in male lower urinary tract. Prostatic smooth muscle tone is decreased by the use of alpha blockers which may lead to improved voiding.*

Phenoxybenzamine

Initial clinical studies showed that non-selective alpha blockers such as phenoxybenzamine, improved symptoms and urinary flow, but were associated with significant side-effects in up to 30% of patients[6]. This led to the introduction of alpha-1 selective blockers.

Alpha-1 selective blockers

Alpha-1 selective blockers, such as prazosin[7], alfuzosin[8] and indoramin[9], and, more recently, the longer-acting alpha-1 selective blockers, such as terazosin, doxazosin, alfuzosin SR (slow release form) and tamsulosin[10], have all been shown to produce improvements in symptom score and in the peak urinary flow rate. Studies have shown a marked improvement in symptoms and peak flow rate with prazosin compared with the placebo, but, in the largest study, there was a high drop-out rate[11] mainly due to dizziness and fatigue.

Interestingly, alpha blockers such as doxazosin appear to reduce blood pressure in hypertensive individuals, but have only minimal effects on blood pressure in normotensive patients. In those 20–30% of patients with BPH who are also hypertensive, alpha blocker therapy may therefore have dual efficacy[12].

Terazosin is one of the most thoroughly evaluated alpha blockers (Figure 6.2). A study in the USA[13] showed a dose-response relationship for a single daily dose (ideally taken at night) and a reasonably low incidence of side-effects. The dose should be titrated up over 1 month from 1 mg/day to a maximum of 5 mg/day. Occasionally patients may need 10 mg/day. The main side-effects were dizziness and tiredness in about 13% of patients. Terazosin resulted in a statistically significant

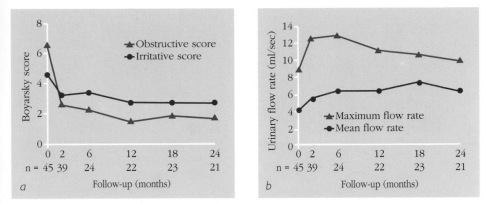

Figure 6.2 *Long-term efficacy of terazosin. (a) Obstructive and irritative Boyarsky symptom scores. (b) Peak and mean urinary flow rates.* Data from Lepor et al. *J Urol* 1992; **147**: 1554.

improvement in both symptom score and maximum and mean urinary flow rate. The efficacy/tolerability ratio of doxazosin appears similar to terazosin[14,15].

Doxazosin. In a recent multicentre study, doxazosin at a final dose of 4 mg/day (after an incremental increase from 1 mg/day) achieved improvements in symptoms and flow rates, together with significant reductions in maximum voiding pressures (Figure 6.3)[14]. Although the usual side-effects associated with alpha blockers (i.e. tiredness, nasal stuffiness and dizziness) were more common, at the end of the trial, many patients opted to stay on medication rather than undergo TURP. As with other alpha blockers, titration of dose improved efficacy, but also increased the incidence of side-effects. Currently, the recommended dose is 4 mg/day, though some patients may benefit from 8 mg/day.

Tamsulosin is a highly selective alpha-1 antagonist, which has been evaluated in a multicentre, randomized, placebo-controlled study[16]. There was a statistically significant improvement in mean urinary flow rate in the treatment group compared with placebo. Tamsulosin, 0.4 mg, resulted in an increase in the peak flow rate of 36%, and a marked symptomatic improvement in 39% of patients.

Alfuzosin. In a randomized placebo-controlled trial, after 6 months,

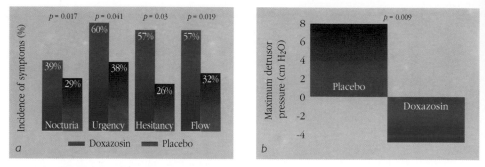

Figure 6.3 *Improvements in (a) symptoms and (b) voiding pressures with doxazosin.* Data from Chapple CR, Carter P, Christmas TJ et al. *J Urol* 1992; **147**: 366A.

symptoms were improved in 82% of patients treated with alfuzosin, 7.5 or 10 mg/day, compared 72% in the placebo group. Nocturnal and diurnal frequencies, hesitancy and urgency decreased significantly after alfuzosin treatment. Peak mean flow rates were significantly higher after 6 weeks of alfuzosin therapy, but there was no significant change in the voided volume. Side-effects, such as dizziness and headaches, tended to be somewhat more severe in alfuzosin-treated patients[8].

Androgen suppression

Agents that suppress androgen stimulation of the prostate can be divided into three groups, namely:

- 5-alpha-reductase inhibitors
- antiandrogens
- luteinizing hormone releasing hormone (LHRH) analogues.

Androgen suppression can also be achieved by the use of progestogen (i.e. antiandrogens), such as megestrol acetate and cyproterone acetate, but these are not widely used in the medical management of BPH.

Mode of action

Most patients with clinical BPH have a considerable increase in the epithelial elements in the transition zone of the prostate gland. The use of androgen-suppressing agents is mainly aimed at this

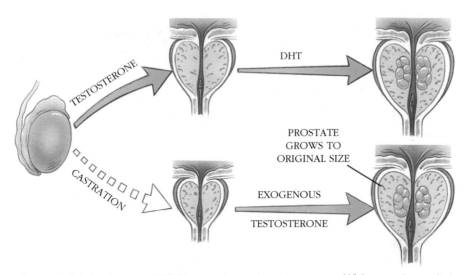

Figure 6.4 *The development of BPH is an androgen-dependent process. While castration results in prostate shrinkage, replacement of androgen drive restores the gland to normal and may permit the development of BPH.*

component, though there is also some stromal reduction, and these drugs probably exert their effect through an overall reduction in prostatic size. The rationale for the use of androgen suppression for BPH is based on a number of observations.

■ Castration or testosterone suppression decreases prostatic volume and symptoms in patients with established BPH (Figure 6.4).

■ Progression to clinical BPH is rare in males castrated before puberty.

■ In males with a congenital deficiency of 5-alpha reductase, the prostate remains underdeveloped, but full sexual function is retained[17].

The conversion of testosterone to dihydrotestosterone (DHT) by 5-alpha reductase is a central part of its intraprostatic metabolism, and inhibition of this enzyme would be expected to cause a regression of BPH (Figure 6.5). The advantage of 5-alpha-reductase inhibitors is that they act without the side-effects associated with other methods of androgen suppression (e.g. impotence, loss of libido, hot flushes and loss of male habitus) because they do not lower serum testosterone.

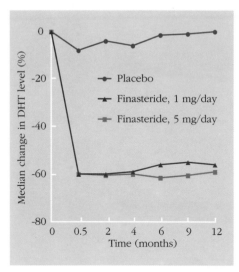

Figure 6.5 *Hormonal effect of finasteride. A rapid decrease in serum dihydrotestosterone (DHT) is achieved and maintained after oral administration.*

5-alpha reductase inhibitors

Finasteride is a 4-azasteroid which has been thoroughly evaluated for efficacy and safety in BPH in many centres throughout the world (Figure 6.6)[18]. The trials have been randomized, placebo-controlled, and continued long-term[19,20]. Most of these studies have concentrated on clinical evaluation by using symptom scores and peak flow rates. The maximum effect of finasteride takes up to 6 months to develop in most patients. Interestingly, a study from Finland showed that positive urodynamic effects take place within 6 months after the introduction of the drug[21]. However, therapy for more than 12 months may be necessary to achieve full urodynamic efficacy[22,23]. Other clinical effects of finasteride that make it a reasonable treatment for symptomatic BPH are presented below.

Finasteride, 5 mg/day, produces a significant and well-maintained improvement in symptom score and peak urinary flow rate compared with placebo (Table 6.4)[19]. A criticism has been that the improvement in peak flow rate, although statistically significant, is still only about 3 ml/second, from about 9 to 12 ml/second (i.e. below the 15 ml/second, empirical cut-off point for 'obstruction'). This flow rate is, however, satisfactory for many patients, and it may be that the high flow rates achieved after surgery are not the priority of most patients. This would seem to be reflected in the improvement in the reasonable symptom scores achieved with finasteride.

Serum PSA values are depressed by about 50% after 6–12 months of finasteride therapy[24] (Figure 6.7). PSA values should therefore be

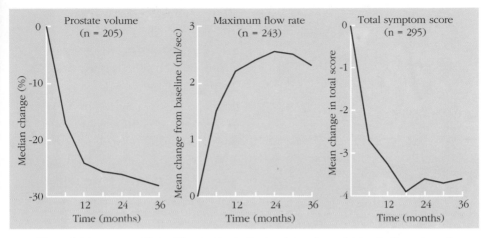

Figure 6.6 *Long-term effects of finasteride. As the prostate volume shrinks, the flow rate and symptom score improve.*

monitored every 6–12 months and any suggestion of a rise in PSA should prompt urological referral for prostatic biopsy.

Prostate volume is reduced by about 30% in two-thirds or more of patients treated with finasteride, and this results in an improvement of symptoms and uroflow.

Side-effects associated with finasteride are rare, the only important one being reduced libido and impotence, which occurs in 3–5% of individuals. Some patients also notice a reduction in ejaculate volume.

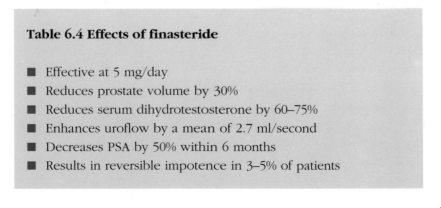

Table 6.4 Effects of finasteride

- Effective at 5 mg/day
- Reduces prostate volume by 30%
- Reduces serum dihydrotestosterone by 60–75%
- Enhances uroflow by a mean of 2.7 ml/second
- Decreases PSA by 50% within 6 months
- Results in reversible impotence in 3–5% of patients

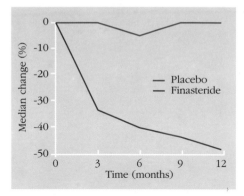

Figure 6.7 *A decrease in PSA values is observed with finasteride therapy.*

These side-effects are reversible on stopping the medication.

Epristeride. Another 5-alpha-reductase inhibitor, epristeride, is also currently being evaluated for activity in BPH. As yet there is little published data available concerning its efficacy and safety, although some useful activity would be anticipated.

Antiandrogens

Flutamide is the main antiandrogen that has been evaluated in the management of BPH[25]; cyproterone acetate and ICI 176334 (Casodex) might also be expected to produce similar effects. However, the randomized and placebo-controlled studies to date have been of short duration and involved relatively small numbers of patients[26]. Although antiandrogens have a positive effect on symptoms and flow, the side-effects of hypogonadism have been prominent. Other side-effects of non-steroidal antiandrogens include impotence/loss of libido, gynaecomastia and diarrhoea. As a result, antiandrogens currently have little significant role to play in the management of symptomatic BPH.

LHRH analogues

LHRH analogues act by inducing reversible chemical castration in patients with symptomatic BPH. Most studies of these agents in BPH have been uncontrolled and performed in small numbers of patients[27], thus limiting any conclusions that can be drawn. Prostatic volume does appear to decrease in patients treated with LHRH analogues, and significant changes in symptom score and peak urinary flow seem to occur. However, the early reports of therapeutic potential for these analogues has not been realized in clinical practice for benign disease.

In addition, LHRH analogues have an unacceptably high level of side-effects which include hot flushes, loss of libido, impotence, loss of facial hair and male habitus. They therefore cannot be recommended at present for the management of symptomatic BPH.

Oestrogen suppression

Mode of action
Oestrogens are almost certainly involved in the pathogenesis of BPH. Testosterone is broken down peripherally by another enzyme (aromatase) to oestradiol and, although the mechanism whereby this metabolic pathway can lead to BPH is not absolutely clear, aromatase inhibitors have been found in experimental and early clinical studies to cause a decrease in prostatic size.

Current investigations
A large clinical trial using the aromatase inhibitor atamestane was recently undertaken. The early results are not, however, encouraging and little improvement in symptom score or peak urinary flow rate has been seen compared with placebo controls.

Phytotherapy
In many countries, plant extracts (Table 6.5), cholesterol-lowering agents, and sundry organ extracts are used in an empirical way to treat the symptoms of prostatism. To date, their clinical value and safety have not been conclusively demonstrated. Most of the clinical trials that have been performed suffer from the criticism that they are short-term and non-placebo controlled, but the small number that have been satisfactory in this manner do not support the view that plant extracts have a major action in relieving either static or dynamic obstruction[28,29]. Until more conclusive evidence is available from placebo-controlled studies, phytotherapeutic agents cannot be considered to have anything more than a placebo action. This does not, however, imply that some patients may not benefit from such a placebo effect.

Table 6.5 Origin of plant extracts used in management of BPH

- *Hypoxis rooperi* (South African star-grass)
- *Urtica* spp. (Stinging nettle)
- *Sabal serrulatum* (Dwarf palm)
- *Serenoa repens B* (American dwarf palm)
- *Cucurbita pepo* (Pumpkin seed)
- *Pygeum africanum* (African plum)
- *Populus tremula* (Aspen)
- *Echinacea purpurea* (Purple coneflower)
- *Secale cereale* (Rye)

Managing prostatitis

Acute prostatitis

The treatment of acute prostatitis is usually straightforward, and all patients should be started on a prolonged course of an antibiotic active against Gram-negative organisms until the culture and sensitivity tests are available. Follow-up cultures must be performed to ensure that complete eradication of the causative organism has occurred. A severe infection may lead to urinary retention which may require suprapubic drainage. Urinary retention usually resolves without the need for further surgical intervention, since the condition responds well to antibiotic therapy. Occasionally, abscess formation occurs and this may rupture spontaneously into the urethra.

Chronic prostatitis

Chronic abacterial prostatitis may respond to anti-inflammatory agents alone, but bacterial prostatic infections require long-term (3-month) courses of antibiotics. Not all antibiotics are, however, capable of achieving satisfactory bactericidal levels within the gland[30,31] and the best agents to use are either the trimethoprim/sulphamethoxazole combination or one of the newer aminoquinolones such as ciprofloxacin or norfloxacin. If this fails, the continuous use of low-dose daily suppressive therapy with an appropriate oral agent, such as nitrofurantoin or trimethoprim plus sulphamethoxazole, may sometimes help. Irritative symptoms may respond to the use of non-steroidal anti-inflammatory drugs (NSAIDs) and anticholinergic drugs.

Following therapy, expressed prostatic secretions (EPS) should become negative on culture and PSA values should fall to within the normal range. Failure of PSA values to decline 3 months after adequate therapy should prompt referral for TRUS-guided prostatic biopsy to exclude prostatic cancer.

Prostatodynia

A trial of alpha-blocking agents or muscle relaxants may sometimes be helpful in treating prostatodynia, but lifestyle changes to reduce stress and anxiety may be more effective. Many of the symptoms are psychogenic rather than physical in nature, and any invasive therapy should generally be avoided

Summary

- Before prescribing medical therapy for BPH, patients should be fully evaluated by symptom score (IPSS), urinary flow rate, DRE, PSA and, ideally, determination of PVR urine volume. Only a full pressure–flow urodynamic study will definitely indicate the presence of obstruction, but it is not practical to perform this test in every patient.

- Patients with mild-to-moderate symptoms of BPH may legitimately be treated by some form of medical treatment, preferably by a 5-alpha-reductase inhibitor or an alpha blocker. Men treated in this way must be carefully followed-up.

■ The other forms of medical treatment such as androgen suppression or aromatase inhibition have not yet been proven in long-term controlled studies to have a significant role in the management of symptomatic BPH, and have a high incidence of side-effects.

■ Plant extracts for BPH probably constitute little more than a relatively expensive means of prescribing placebo.

References

1   Mebust WK, Holtgrewe HL, Cockett ATK, Peters PC. Transurethral prostatectomy: immediate and postoperative complications. A cooperative study of 13 participating institutions evaluating 3885 patients. *J Urol* 1989; **141**: 243–8.

2   Roos NP, Wennberg JE, Malenka DJ *et al.* Mortality and reoperation after open and transurethral resection of the prostate for benign prostatic hyperplasia. *N Engl J Med* 1989; **320**: 1120–4.

3   Garraway WM, Collins GN, Lee RJ. High prevalence of benign prostatic hypertrophy in the community. *Lancet* 1991; **488**: 469–71.

4   Wennberg JE, Mulley AF, Hanley D *et al.* An assessment of prostatectomy for benign urinary tract obstruction. Geographic variations and the evaluation of medical outcomes. *JAMA* 1988; **259**: 3027–30.

5   Shapiro E, Lepor H. Alpha adrenergic receptors in hyperplasic human prostate: identification and characterization using ^{3}H rauwolsine. *J Urol* 1992; **135**: 1038–41.

6   Caine M, Perlerg S, Meretyk S. A placebo-controlled double-blind study of the effect of phenoxybenzamine in benign prostatic obstruction. *Br J Urol* 1978; **50**: 551–4.

7   Hedlund H, Andersson KE. Effects of prazosin in patients with benign prostatic obstruction. *J Urol* 1983; **130**: 275–8.

8   Jardin A, Bensadoun H, Delauche-Cavallier MC, Attali P, BPH-ALF group. Alfuzosin for the treatment of benign prostatic hypertrophy. *Lancet* 1991; **337**: 1457–61.

9   Stott MA, Abrams P. Indoramin in the treatment of prostatic bladder outflow obstruction. *Br J Urol* 1991; **67**: 499–501.

10   Kawabe K, Niijima T. Use of an alpha blocker YM-12617 in micturition difficulty. *Urol Int* 1987; **42**: 280–4.

11   Kirby RS, Coppinger SWC, Corcoran MO, Chapple CR, Flannigan M, Milroy EJG. Prazosin in the treatment of prostatic obstruction. A placebo controlled study. *Br J Urol* 1987; **60**: 136–42.

12   Kirby RS, Chapple CR, Christmas TJ. Doxazosin: minimal blood pressure effects in normotensive BPH patients. *J Urol* 1993; **149**: 434A.

13 Lepor H, Auerbach S, Puras-Baez A *et al*. A randomised, placebo-controlled multicentre study of the efficacy and safety of terazosin in the treatment of benign prostatic hyperplasia. *J Urol* 1992; **148**: 1467–74.

14 Chapple CR, Christmas TJ, Milroy EJG, Abrams P, Kirby RS. A three month placebo-controlled study of doxazosin on prostatic outflow obstruction. *J Urol* 1992; **147:** 366A.

15 Christensen MM, Holme JB, Rasmussen PC *et al*. Doxazosin treatment in patients with prostatic obstruction. A double-blind placebo-controlled study. *Scan J Urol Nephrol* 1993; **27**: 39–44.

16 Kawabe K, Veno A, Takimoto Y, Aso Y, Kato H. Use of an alpha-blocker, YM 617, in the treatment of benign prostatic hypertrophy. YM 617 Clinical Study Group. *J Urol* 1990; **144**: 908–12.

17 Imperato-McGinley J, Guevro L, Gauteri T, Petersen RE. Steroid 5-alpha-reductase deficiency in a man: an inherited form of pseudohermaphroditism. *Science* 1974; **186**: 1213–15.

18 Stoner E. The clinical effects of a 5-alpha reductase inhibitor, finasteride, on benign prostatic hyperplasia. *J Urol* 1992; **147**: 1298–302.

19 Gormley GJ, Stoner E, Bruskewitz RC *et al*. The effect of finasteride in men with benign prostatic 29 hyperplasia. *N Engl J Med* 1992; **327**: 1185–91.

20 Finasteride Study Group. Finasteride (MK-906) in the treatment of benign prostatic hyperplasia. *Prostate* 1993; **22**: 291–9.

21 Tammela TLJ, Konturri MJ. Urodynamic effects of finasteride in the treatment of bladder outlet obstruction due to benign prostatic hyperplasia. *J Urol* 1993; **149:** 342–4.

22 Kirby RS, Vale J, Bryan J, Holmes K, Webb JAW. Long-term urodynamic effects of finasteride in benign prostatic hyperplasia: a pilot study. *Eur Urol* 1993; **24**: 20–6

23 Kirby RS, Bryan J, Christmas TJ, Vale J, Eardley I, Webb J. Finasteride in the management of benign prostatic hyperplasia – a urodynamic study. *Br J Urol* 1992; **70**: 65–72.

24 Guess HA, Heyse JF, Gormley GJ. The effect of finasteride on prostate specific antigen in men with benign prostatic hyperplasia. *Prostate* 1993; **22**: 31–7.

25 Stone NN. Flutamide in the treatment of benign prostatic hypertrophy. *Urology* 1989; **34**: 64–9.

26 Wolf H, Madsen P. Treatment of benign prostatic hypertrophy with progestational agents: a preliminary report. *J Urol* 1968; **99**: 790–5.

27 Peters CA, Walsh PC. The effect of nafarelin acetate, a luteinizing hormone releasing hormone agonist, on benign prostatic hyperplasia. *N Eng J Med* 1987; **317**: 599–604.

28 Champault G, Patel JC, Bonnard AM. A double-blind trial of an extract of the plant *Serenoa repens* in benign prostatic hyperplasia. *Br J Clin Pharmacol* 1984; **18**: 461–2.

29 Reece-Smith H, Memon A, Smart CJ, Dewbury K. The value of permixon in benign prostatic hypertrophy. *Br J Urol* 1986; **58:** 36–40.

30 Stamey TA, Meares EM, Winningham DG. Chronic bacterial prostatitis and the diffusion of drugs into prostatic fluid. *J Urol* 1970; **103**: 187–94.

31 Naber KG. Use of quinolones in urinary tract infections and prostatitis. *Rev Infect Dis* 1989; **11 (suppl 5)**; S1321–37.

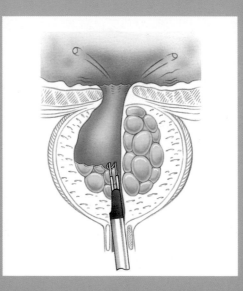

Chapter 7

Specialist management of BPH

Although the use of technological intervention and surgery in the treatment of benign prostatic hyperplasia (BPH) falls into the domain of the urologist, it is important that family practitioners become acquainted and keep up to date with the options available (Table 7.1). In addition to standard surgical approaches that still constitute the mainstay of treatment for most patients with BPH, new treatment options are being introduced at an unparalleled rate. Increasingly well-informed patients are now requesting information about these new treatment methods, not all of which have lived up to the 'hype' that has surrounded their launch.

Technological interventional methods

Many attempts, using a variety of new technologies, are being made to develop the 'ideal' interventional treatment for symptomatic BPH; there is a great enthusiasm on the part of urologists to do so. Most of these techniques are aimed at reducing the 'static' element of outflow obstruction – the transition zone volume. All aim to achieve a satisfactory long-term therapeutic effect with fewer complications, lower costs, and a shorter hospital stay than traditional surgery.

However, as yet, none of the new minimally invasive procedures to arise has been judged to have replaced transurethral resection of

Table 7.1 Specialist treatments for BPH

Technological intervention
- Balloon dilatation
- Prostatic stents (temporary and permanent)
- Hyperthermia
- Thermotherapy
- Laser ablation
- High-intensity focused ultrasound
- Focused extracorporeal pyrotherapy
- Transurethral needle ablation (TUNA)

Surgery
- Open prostatectomy
- Transurethral resection of the prostate (TURP)
- Transurethral incision of the prostate (TUIP)

the prostate (TURP) when stringent outcome criteria have been applied. While the prospects of these techniques in the management of BPH are exciting, it is important that their longer-term clinical value and safety are assessed at an early stage, in order that their place in the ever-expanding therapeutic armamentarium of this disease becomes clear.

Balloon dilatation
The rationale for the use of balloon dilatation (Figure 7.1) is that it splits the prostatic urethra in the form of an anterior commissurotomy. Although a laudable aim, the reality is that splitting rather than incising the prostate is neither theoretically sound nor practically very effective. The idea was introduced last century by the early urological surgeons and has been popularized in modern times by Burhenne[1].

Balloon dilatation has been evaluated in a number of centres[2], but has, at no stage, gained general acceptance among urologists. Although some studies have shown that balloon dilatation provided a symptomatic improvement[3], other studies have shown a large associated placebo effect and no difference between balloon dilatation and the passage of a cystoscope[4]; in fact one study showed that balloon dilatation did not cause any decrease in the urodynamic changes of obstruction[5].

The most recent study has, however, shown that in small numbers and a short-term evaluation, balloon dilatation of the prostate yields results that are comparable to TURP. Unfortunately, these results have not been found in other centres, and so most urologists still feel that balloon dilatation of the prostate has little if any role in the management of BPH[6]. As it requires an anaesthetic, and its long-term outcome is unclear, it is very unlikely that it will displace TURP in the management of symptomatic BPH.

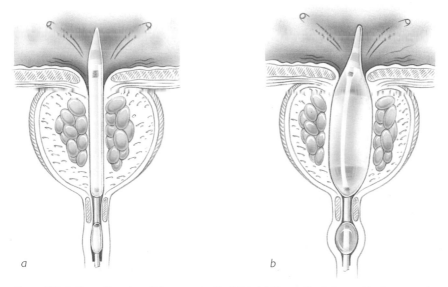

a   b

Figure 7.1 *Balloon dilatation of the prostate for BPH. (a) The device is located in the prostatic urethra by palpation of the balloon in the bulbar urethra. (b) The 90F balloon is then inflated to dilate the prostatic urethra.*

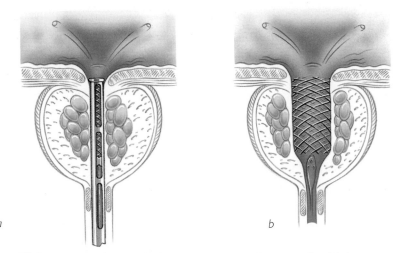

a　　　　　　　　　　　　　　　　　　　　*b*

Figure 7.2 *Prostatic stent for BPH. (a) Cystoscopic insertion of an expanding 'Urolume' stainless steel prostatic stent. (b) The open stent maintains patency of the prostatic urethra and gradually epithelializes.*

Prostatic stents

The concept of a metal spiral stent (Figure 7.2) inserted into the prostatic urethra to relieve symptoms in patients with prostatic enlargement was originally introduced by Fabian in 1980. The success of the spiral stent in the management of urethral strictures encouraged researchers to investigate its use in the management of prostatic enlargement. Today, however, associated complications have limited the role of stents to the treatment of patients with acute or chronic urinary retention who are unable to withstand a surgical procedure such as prostatectomy. Currently available prostatic stents may be either temporary or permanent.

Temporary stents, such as the gold-plated Prostakath, the Nissenkorn intraurethral catheter and the more recent thermo-expandable Memokath, are associated with complications such as displacement and encrustation. They can be inserted cystoscopically or under local anaesthetic using transrectal ultrasound guidance.

When used in patients with acute or chronic urinary retention who are unsuitable for surgery, these minimally invasive procedures are associated with a marked improvement in flow rate. However, associated complications, such as encrustation and migration, and the necessity for the device to be replaced at 6-monthly intervals has limited their role in the treatment of symptomatic BPH[7].

Permanent stents, such as the Urolume™ [8] and the titanium ASI 'Titan'™ stent[9] can also be introduced relatively easily and expand to fit the contours of the prostatic urethra. Again, these stents are associated with an excellent relief of obstruction in acute urinary retention, but only a modest longer-term improvement in flow rate and symptom score in patients with symptomatic BPH who do not present with retention. They are also subject to a number of complications, such as encrustation, and hyperplasia of the prostatic urothelium through the holes in the mesh. Patients may also complain of urethral pain and irritation, which currently limits their use to only a minority of individuals with outflow obstruction due to BPH who are unfit for conventional surgery.

Heat treatment

The idea that local heat will cure prostatic disease has been the source of sporadic interest since the 18th century. With current enthusiasm for new technology, this theory is enjoying something of a renaissance. Heat treatment for patients with symptomatic BPH is based on the concept that a transrectal probe with rectal protection is capable of reducing bladder outflow obstruction. Hyperthermia implies an intraprostatic temperature of 41–45°C, and this, and the higher temperatures within adenomas produced by 'thermotherapy' (45–55°C), have been the focus of many recent studies.

Transrectal and transurethral hyperthermia. Several hyperthermia machines, which use microwave technology to heat the prostate, for example the Prostathermer and Primus (transrectal), and the Thermex II and BSD Prostate machine (transurethral), are all capable of producing an intraprostatic temperature of about 42–44°C (Figure 7.3). Early reports have indicated improvements in peak urinary flow rate and symptom score in about 45% of patients[10]. The group recommended for treatment was, however, fairly restricted, comprising patients with small prostates and only mild-to-moderate symptoms.

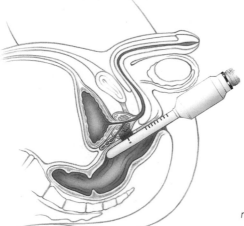

Figure 7.3 *Transrectal hyperthermia. The microwave delivery device is passed per rectum and microwave energy directed anteriorly.*

Other studies followed, and an improvement in both symptom scores and flow rates has been reported using transurethral hyperthermia[11].

However, in a recent multicentre sham-controlled study of transrectal and transurethral hyperthermia performed in Paris, France, no difference between a sham procedure and treatment with hyperthermia in either subjective or objective criteria was observed, except at 1 year when symptom scores in the treatment group were marginally superior[12]. These results have placed the future of hyperthermia in the management of patients with symptomatic BPH in some doubt, and the technique cannot be generally recommended at present.

Thermotherapy or transurethral microwave therapy, is delivered by the Prostatron™ (Figure 7.4), which has been extensively evaluated in many centres worldwide. Thermotherapy uses a combination of transurethrally administered heat energy and conductive cooling. The cooling is supposed to prevent urethral damage and pain. The prostatic tissue itself is subjected to a temperature of 45–55°C; these higher temperatures may induce tissue necrosis and possibly induce damage to the intraprostatic nerves and alpha receptors. Several studies have shown significant improvements in symptom scores and peak urinary flow rates using the Prostatron[13].

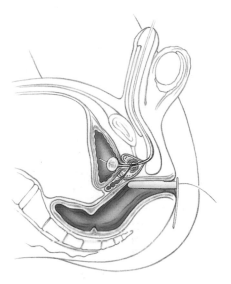

Figure 7.4 *Transurethral microwave thermotherapy (TUMT). The 'Prostatron' microwave delivery catheter is passed per urethra and located in the prostatic urethra by inflation of the catheter balloon. Rectal temperature is monitored by means of a device inserted into the rectum.*

Recent sham studies[14] suggest that thermotherapy exerts a measurable effect on the prostate which is more than placebo. A review of many European studies into the use of thermotherapy shows that there is a reasonably long-lasting improvement in peak flow rate of approximately 3 ml/second[15]. Although there is no major difference between these results and those achieved with medical treatment of BPH, there is no question that thermotherapy is capable of producing some effect on the prostate. Although the improvements in symptom scores and peak urinary flow rates are not comparable with TURP, continued studies with increased energy delivery are justified. One important disadvantage of the Prostatron, however, is that 25% of patients experience temporary acute urinary retention after therapy[16].

Laser treatment

Laser technology has been used with increasing enthusiasm in the management of BPH in a number of urological centres (Figure 7.5). Among its potential advantages are an absence of postoperative bleeding, and a minimal in-patient hospital stay.

Although a number of different types of laser energy have been used, the most popular at present is the neodymium-YAG laser. The

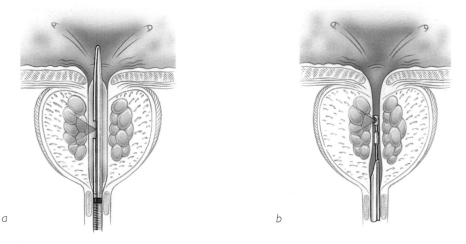

Figure 7.5 *(a) The TULIP transurethral delivery system. The in-built ultrasound system allows precise visualization of the treated area. (b) Endoscopic laser ablation of the prostate. The side-firing delivery probe is inserted through a cystoscope and laser energy applied to the adenoma tissue under vision.*

laser can be applied either under ultrasound guidance, as in transurethral laser incision of the prostate (TULIP) or under endoscopic control as in endoscopic laser ablation of the prostate (ELAP). It can be fired at a distance from or directly in contact with prostatic tissue; it can also be introduced by a needle or fibre into the interstitium of the prostate. Many researchers believe laser technology may be one of the treatments of the future for prostatic disease, and two recent studies from the USA have shown a 68% improvement in symptom scores and a 78% improvement in peak flow rates. These results are encouraging, but more formal comparisons with TURP are needed, in large numbers of patients with a long-term outcome evaluation[17,18].

Although the procedure itself is not excessively traumatic for the patient, it must be performed under some form of anaesthesia. The necessity to stay in hospital is governed by the urologist or patient preference; it is now often offered to the patient as a day-case operation.

The technology is expensive – a laser may cost more than US$100,000 and the laser-deflecting fibres US$500 each. Cost constraints may therefore limit the extensive use of this technology in many units.

Complications. Laser ablation of the prostate occurs at a higher temperature than hyperthermia or thermotherapy. This causes coagulative necrosis of the prostate and subsequent passage of slough. This slough and swelling in response to heat damage is sometimes a problem and, in the immediate postoperative period, most patients have some difficulties in passing urine, as well as some quite persistent perineal and urethral pain. This is managed by a suprapubic or urethral catheter, which must often be left in place for 5 days and sometimes longer.

Latest techniques and developments

New methods of supplying greater degrees of heat to the prostate, and yet preserving the integrity of the surrounding tissues have been introduced. All of these are at an early stage of development and are undergoing extensive studies to evaluate their effectiveness and safety, and also to assess potential complications. These techniques are of considerable interest and may well herald a new dawn not only in the management of BPH, but also prostate cancer.

High-intensity focused ultrasound causes tissue ablation by inducing high temperatures (90–100°C) in tissues not in contact with, and in fact some distance from, the probe[19]. Thus by inserting a probe into the rectum, high temperatures can be induced in the prostate without damaging the wall of the rectum.

Early clinical studies found that high-intensity focused ultrasound produced symptomatic improvement and an increase in the peak urinary flow rate, though the number of patients treated was relatively small. This has been confirmed by the early results of a more recent study in a large number of patients over a longer period. In a recent study[20], the peak flow rate had improved at 3 months from a mean of 9 ml/second to 14.4 ml/second, with a corresponding decrease in post-void residual urine (PVR) and a highly significant improvement in symptom score.

Other independent experimental studies, using a different system, but the same principle of high-intensity focused ultrasound, have shown that this technique causes lesions in the prostate[21] (Figure 7.6);

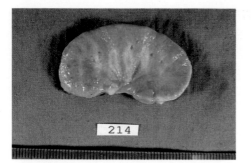

Figure 7.6 *Lesions to the prostate caused by high-intensity focused ultrasound.*

controlled clinical studies into this machine will follow in due course.

Focused extracorporeal pyrotherapy delivers ultrashort waves to the prostate extra-corporeally rather than trans-rectally[22]. Although this has exciting possibilities in the management of urological cancer, its use in symptomatic BPH is at present limited by the fact that it is focused on the prostate by ultrasound. Transabdominal ultrasound can visualize only the middle lobe of the prostate reliably and so, unless the prostate has a large median lobe, this form of treatment will be inappropriate. However, many new areas of development are being explored, and interesting possibilities may lie ahead.

Transurethral needle ablation (TUNA) using radio waves delivers high temperatures (120°C) to the prostate transurethrally,

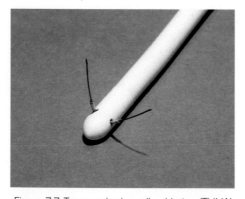

Figure 7.7 *Transurethral needle ablation (TUNA) of the prostate uses radiofrequency antennae to deliver high temperatures to the prostate without anaesthesia.*

without an anaesthetic and with minimal disruption to the prostatic urethra (Figure 7.7). The effects of TUNA are demonstrable both histologically and by magnetic resonance imaging (MRI) and have been corroborated in clinical studies showing marked increases in urinary flow rates from 9 ml/second to as high as 17 ml/second. An international trial into the use of this technique is currently being undertaken and the results of this are keenly awaited.

Watchful waiting

Is it reasonable to defer treatment in patients with symptoms of prostatism, by so-called 'watchful waiting'? Under some circumstances, the answer to this is yes. Provided that the patient with mild symptoms has been adequately assessed, and does not have a malignant prostate, a careful period of watchful waiting may well be indicated. Watchful waiting should not be a byword for neglect and it is clearly not an option for those patients who do not wish to tolerate bothersome symptoms any longer or those with absolute indications for surgery (Table 7.2).

Table 7.2 Absolute indications for surgery

- Recurrent episodes of haematuria
- Recurrent attacks of urinary infection
- Acute or chronic retention of urine
- Bladder stones secondary to BPH
- Upper tract dilatation
- Large diverticula

Surgical options

TURP is by far the most common procedure used (representing about 95% of prostate operations), though open retropubic prostatectomy may be more appropriate for very large prostates (> 100 g). When the prostate is small and yet is the cause of outflow obstruction and associated perhaps with an obstructive bladder neck, the procedure of choice could well be a transurethral incision of the prostate (TUIP).

Open prostatectomy

Open prostatectomy is performed through a lower abdominal incision, either mid-line or transverse suprapubic, and either through the bladder (transvesical prostatectomy) or through the capsule of the

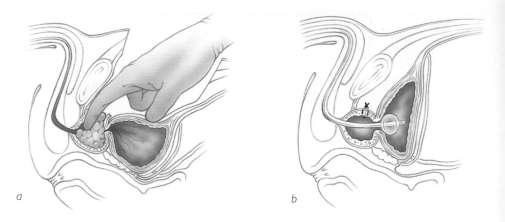

Figure 7.8 *Millin's retropubic prostatectomy. (a) An incision is made through the anterior prostatic capsule and the transition zone adenoma enucleated by means of finger dissection. (b) The capsule is closed and a Foley catheter is retained for 5 days.*

prostate (Millin's prostatectomy). In both cases, the adenoma is enucleated and a urethral catheter is left draining the bladder for up to 5 days postoperatively. The wound usually heals quickly and is not excessively painful (Figure 7.8). The procedure is especially suitable for those patients with large adenomas (> 100 g).

Open prostatectomy is a very effective method of treating benign

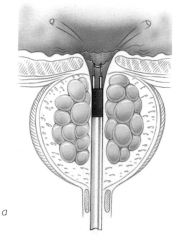

Figure 7.9 *Transurethral resection of the prostate (TURP). (a) The median lobe is resected by a resectoscope. (b) Further tissue is then resected until all the transitional adenoma is removed. (c) A 'cavity' persists which tends to shrink with time.*

a

prostatic obstruction; symptoms improve markedly and the mean peak flow usually increases to more than 20 ml/second postoperatively. Furthermore, the likelihood of patients requiring further surgery is lower with open prostatectomy than with TURP[23]. However, the procedure is more invasive and requires longer hospitalization than transurethral surgery, which makes it very much less attractive to informed patients.

Transurethral resection of the prostate

TURP is an operation which has become increasingly refined over the last 50 years (Figure 7.9). With the optical systems that are now available, it can be carried out using a visual display on a video screen. The procedure has become relatively easy to perform in experienced hands, but should be undertaken only by surgeons who have specifically trained in the technique.

TURP is carried out through a resectoscope with a diathermy loop. Slivers of tissue are excised and then evacuated through the resectoscope sheath. Spinal epidural or light general anaesthesia is usually used and the patient will require a urinary catheter for 36–48 hours postoperatively. Postoperative pain is not usually a problem, symptoms rapidly improve and peak urinary flow rates generally increase to above 18–20 ml/second.

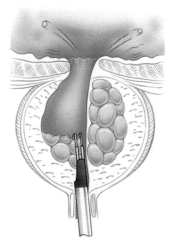

b

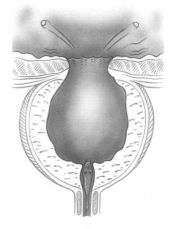

c

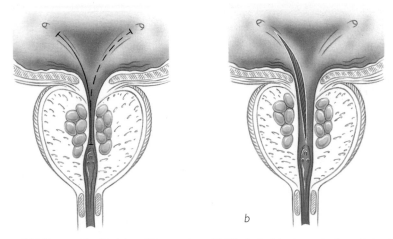

a   b

Figure 7.10 *Transurethral incision of the prostate (TUIP). An incision is made through the bladder neck area (a) allowing the lateral tissue areas to spring apart (b). Some urologists use a bilateral incision, as shown.*

Transurethral incision of the prostate

TUIP is a simple procedure which has been practised since the last century (Figure 7.10). With advances in optic technology, it is now very simple and straightforward. TUIP is, however, suitable only for small prostates with a high bladder neck and no middle lobe enlargement. An incision is made from just below the ureteric orifice on one or both sides and carried through the bladder neck to 0.1 cm proximal to the verumontanum. The results are generally excellent, with a postoperative peak flow rate of about 18 ml/second[24]. The incidence of complications is very low, and even retrograde ejaculation occurs in no more than 10% of patients. A proportion of patients, however, do not improve or subsequently relapse, and may then need a TURP.

Complications of TURP (Table 7.3)

Primary haemorrhage, which occurs within 24 hours of surgery and is directly related to the surgery itself, is not usually severe. A blood transfusion is necessary in only 5–15 % of patients and hence the policy is to not cross match the patient's blood before TURP.

Table 7.3 Outcome of surgical treatment for BPH

Outcome	TUIP	TURP	Open prostatectomy
Likelihood of symptom improvement	80%	88%	98%
Reduction in symptom score	73%	85%	79%
Improvement in mean peak flow rate	8–15 ml/sec	8–18 ml/sec	8–23 ml/sec
Likelihood of further treatment within 5 years	8.1%	3.4%	0.4%
Complications			
Overall rate	14%	16.1%	21.7%
Risk of blood transfusion	2%	5–15%	30%
Incontinence	0.1%	0.8%	0.4%
Erectile impotence	12.6%	15.7%	19.0%
Retrograde ejaculation	10%	68%	72%
Need for operative treatment of surgical complications	2.9%	3.3%	4.2%
Likelihood of death within 90 days of surgery	< 1%	1.5%	2%

Clearly if there is a predisposition to haemorrhage, this would need to be investigated and appropriate steps taken. Many patients who have had heart valve surgery or myocardial ischaemia and are on warfarin undergo TURP. The warfarin must be stopped 4–5 days preoperatively and cover continued with intravenous heparin. Heparin is stopped 4 hours preoperatively and reintroduced postoperatively. Patients with a history of ischaemic heart disease may be taking aspirin, which should also be stopped 2 weeks before surgery.

Secondary haemorrhage after TURP is often handled by the family practitioner. It generally occurs 10–14 days postoperatively and is a relatively common, if minor, occurrence. The patient should be advised to rest in bed, increase his fluid intake, and take appropriate antibiotics depending on urine culture and sensitivity reports. Occasionally secondary haemorrhage can be severe; if clot retention supervenes the patient will require hospitalization and catheterization, and occasionally bladder washout to help remove the clots.

Urinary incontinence after TURP is most commonly due to pre-existent detrusor instability with or without sphincter weakness. Urge incontinence is most characteristic, and will usually disappear within a few weeks or months after surgery. Urge incontinence is best treated with anticholinergics, which will, of course, also treat the symptoms of frequency and nocturia.

Occasionally stress incontinence can occur, which is due to some degree of sphincter damage. Stress incontinence will also usually disappear with time, but if after 6 months residual stress incontinence is concerning the patient, the insertion of an artificial urinary sphincter may be occasionally necessary.

Urethral stricture is a very disappointing complication of TURP for both patient and surgeon, which can occur in up to 5–6% of cases[25]. Common sites are the external urethral meatus, the bladder neck, the peno-scrotal junction, and the bulbar urethra. The incidence of strictures after TURP can be minimized by urethrotomy or careful gauging of the size of the urethra with Clutton's sounds, and the use of a resectoscope which will fit easily within the well-lubricated urethra. Urethral strictures most commonly present 4–5 months after surgery in patients who have, up to that time, had great relief of their preoperative symptoms and are usually disappointed at the sudden change in events, when symptoms of outflow obstruction return.

Initial treatment is most commonly direct vision internal urethrotomy. If the stricture is at the meatus, gentle meatal dilatation may be sufficient. Occasionally, optical urethrotomy or reconstructive surgery of the urethra may be required.

Sexual dysfunction. Retrograde ejaculation is the most common sexual dysfunction following prostatectomy (Figure 7.11). The incidence after TURP and open prostatectomy is about 70%, though only 10% following TUIP. Every patient who is undergoing prostatic surgery

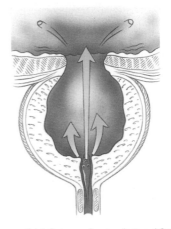

Figure 7.11 Retrograde ejaculation. After transurethral resection of the prostate (TURP), semen passes retrogradely into the bladder at the time of orgasm because of the loss of the bladder neck sphincter mechanism.

should, of course, be warned that retrograde ejaculation may occur. Most patients who have been properly informed are not troubled by retrograde ejaculation in the longer term.

Some patients complain of impotence after prostatic surgery. While there is no clear surgical explanation for this, the cavernous nerves and vessels do pass near the apex of the gland. It is worth remembering that in middle-aged and elderly men, pre-existing impotence, either psychogenic or physically based, may be present. If the patient wishes, impotence can be treated by intracorporeal injections of papaverine and phentolamine, or prostaglandin E_1. The use of implantable penile prostheses and the vacuum pump are also acceptable forms of therapy for some patients.

Outcome of TURP

While most patients who have had a TURP are satisfied with the outcome, recent studies have shown that 15–20% have a less than perfect result[26]. These findings may reflect the present non-selective policy for TURP, whereby patient selection is generally based on their symptoms which are nonspecific; sometimes the flow rate may not be absolutely selective either. In addition, patients do not always describe their symptoms or their effect on quality of life as thoroughly to the urologist as they do to their family practitioner. Although recent retrospective studies have shown that there is a higher re-operation rate in patients undergoing TURP than in those undergoing open prostatectomy[23], this does not justify an abandonment of the less invasive procedure. The reduction of symptom score and improvement in peak urinary flow rate is greater with either TURP or open prostatectomy than any other currently available therapy for BPH.

Although TURP is a satisfactory and relatively safe method for treating prostatic outflow obstruction, it has been argued that, in the future, more careful evaluation of the impact of the symptoms and the presence of obstruction is required before such surgery is undertaken. This will ensure that only those patients who are genuinely bothered by true bladder outflow obstruction will be subjected to prostatic surgery, and this, in turn, may enhance the results obtained (Table 7.3).

Mortality after TURP in the best centres is now less than 0.3%[27], but retrospective studies of cases at all units suggest an overall mortality of about 1.5%[23]. Many patients undergoing prostatectomy have some co-morbid condition and this is definitely related to postoperative mortality. Serious postoperative sepsis has been virtually eradicated by the use of antibiotic prophylaxis.

Balance-sheet concept and patient-based decisions

Because there are insufficient efficacy, safety and outcome data to tailor any particular therapy to each individual patient, the 'balance-sheet' concept may be helpful (Figure 7.12). This involves explaining to the patient that treatment results in both indirect and direct health outcomes. The indirect health outcomes may be of no consequence to the patient's mind (e.g. improvements in flow rate, PVR urine and pressure flow studies), while the direct health outcome, that is improvement in symptoms, is extremely important. In order that the patient can make a fully informed decision, the positive effects, the likelihood of successful long-term outcome and the relative incidence

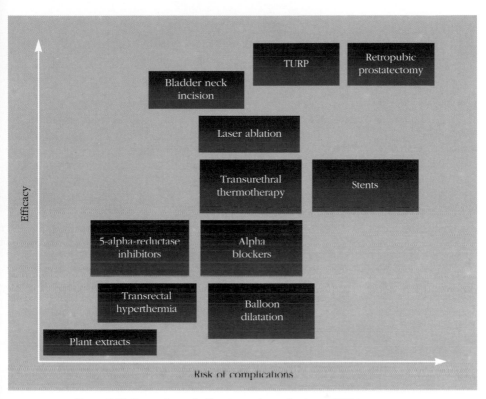

Figure 7.12 *Comparison of efficacies and complications of BPH treatments.*

of complications for every treatment option must be explained fully.

The importance of a patient-based decision cannot be over-estimated. Patient counselling may be helped by the recent introduction of interactive videodiscs and other visual materials which explain the condition and the treatment options. This may allow a shared decision between patient, family practitioner and urologist based on understanding of anatomy, pathology, and treatment.

Summary

■ Acute and chronic retention of urine remain absolute indications for prostate surgery.

■ For patients with symptomatic BPH who do not have acute or chronic urinary retention, it is advisable to have a full informed discussion to balance the risks against the benefits of surgery.

■ The technological approaches other than TURP for the treatment of symptomatic BPH are currently being investigated in multicentre trials throughout the world. At present, their cost-effectiveness and longer-term efficacy in relieving symptoms and bladder outflow obstruction is under careful scrutiny. As yet, none of the newer technologies has been found to be superior in efficacy to TURP.

References

1 Burhenne HJ, Chisholm RJ, Quenville NF. Prostatic hyperplasia; radiological intervention. *Radiology* 1987; **152**: 655–7.

2 Wasserman NF, Reddy PK, Zhang F, Berg PA. Experimental treatment of benign prostatic hyperplasia with transurethral balloon dilatation of the prostate: a preliminary study in 73 humans. *Radiology* 1990; **177**: 485–94.

3 Dowd JB, Smith JJ. Balloon dilatation of the prostate. *Urol Clin North Am* 1990; **17**: 671–7.

4 Lepor H, Sypherd R, Derus J, Machi G. A randomised double-blind study comparing the efficacy of cystoscopy versus balloon dilatation of the prostate in males with symptomatic benign prostatic hyperplasia. *J Urol* 1991; **145**: 362A.

5 McLoughlin J, Keane DF, Jager R, Gill KP, Machann L, Williams G. Dilatation of the prostate with a 35mm balloon. *Br J Urol* 1991; **67**: 177–81.

6 Vale JA, Miller PD, Kirby RS. Balloon dilatation of the prostate: should it have a place in the urologist's armamentarium? *J Royal Soc Med* 1993; **86**: 83–6.

7 Nordling J, Oversen H, Poulsen AL. Intraprostatic spiral: clinical results in 150 consecutive patients. *J Urol* 1992; **147**: 645–7.

8 Chapple CR, Milroy EJG, Rickards D. Permanently implanted urethral stent for prostatic obstruction in the unfit patient. *Br J Urol* 1990; **66**: 58–65.

9 Kirby RS, Heard SR, Miller PD *et al.* Use of the ASI titanium stent in the management of bladder outflow obstruction due to benign prostatic hyperplasia. *J Urol* 1992; **148**: 1195–7.

10 Zerbib M, Conquy S, Steg A, Martinache PR, Flam T, Fabre B. Localized transrectal hyperthermia in the treatment of obstructive manifestations of prostatic adenoma. Review of the literature and personal experience. *J Urol* 1992; **98**: 89–92.

11 Devonec M, Ogden C, Perrin P, Carter S. Clinical response to transurethral microwave thermotherapy is thermal dose-dependent. *Eur Urol* 1993; **23**: 267–74.

12 Cockett ATK, Khoury S, Aso Y, Chatelain C, Denis L, Griffiths K, Murphy G, eds. *2nd International Consultation on Benign Prostatic Hyperplasia.* Paris: SCI, 1994; 460.

13 De La Rosette JJ, Frøehling FM, Debruyne FM. Clinical results with microwave thermotherapy of benign prostatic hyperplasia. *Eur Urol* 1993; **23**: 68–71.

14 Ogden CW, Reddy P, Johnson H, Ramsay JWA, Carter S. Sham versus transurethral microwave thermotherapy in patients with symptoms of benign prostatic bladder outflow obstruction. *Lancet* 1993; **341**: 14–17.

15 Cockett ATK, Khoury S, Aso Y, Chatelain C, Denis L, Griffiths K, Murphy G, eds. *2nd International Consultation on Benign Prostatic Hyperplasia.* Paris: SCI, 1994: 453–506.

16 Kirby RS, Williams G, Witherow R, Milroy EJG, Philp T. The Prostatron transurethral microwave device in the treatment of bladder outflow obstruction due to BPH. *Br J Urol* 1993; **72**: 190–4.

17 McCullough DL, Roth RA, Babayan RK, Poidon JO, Reese JH, Crawford ED. Transurethral ultrasound guided laser induced prostatectomy. *J Urol* 1993; **150**: 1607.

18 Norris JP, Norris Dm, Lee RD, Rubenstein MA. Visual laser ablation of the prostate: clinical experience in 108 patients. *J Urol* 1993; **150**: 1612–14.

19 Ter Haar G, Rivens I, Chien L, Riddler S. High intensity focused ultrasound for the treatment of rat tumours. *Phys Med Biol* 1991; **36**: 1495–1501.

20 Madersbarcher S, Kratzik C, Szabo N, Susani M, Vingers J, Marberger M. Tissue ablation in benign prostatic hyperplasia with high intensity focused ultrasound. *Eur Urol* 1993; **23**: 39–43.

21 Gelet A, Chapelon JY, Margonari J *et al.* High intensity focussed ultrasound experimentation on human benign prostatic hyperplasia. *Eur Urol* 1993; **23**: 44–7.

22 Vallancien G, Chartier-Kastler E, Bataille N, Chopin D, Harouni M, Bougaran J. Focused extracorporeal pyrotherapy. *Eur Urol* 1993; **23**: 48–52.

23 Roos NP, Wennberg JE, Malenka DJ, Fisher ES, McPherson K, Anderson TF. Mortality and re-operation after open and trans-urethral resection of the prostate for benign prostatic hyperplasia. *N Engl J Med* 1989; **320**: 1120–4.

24 Orandi A. Transurethral incision of the prostate compared with transurethral resection of the prostate in matching cases. *J Urol* 1987; **138**: 810–15.

25 Lentz MC, Mebust WK, Foret JD, Melchior J. Urethral strictures following transurethral prostatectomy a review of 223 resections. *J Urol* 1977; **117**: 194–6.

26 Neal DE, Ramsden PD, Sharples L, Smith A, Powell PH, Styles RA. Outcome of prostatectomy. *BMJ* 1989; **299**: 762–7.

27 Mebust WK, Holtgrewe HL, Cockett ATK, Peters PC. Transurethral prostatectomy: immediate and postoperative complications. A cooperative study of 13 participating institutions evaluating 3885 patients. *J Urol* 1989; **141**: 243–8.

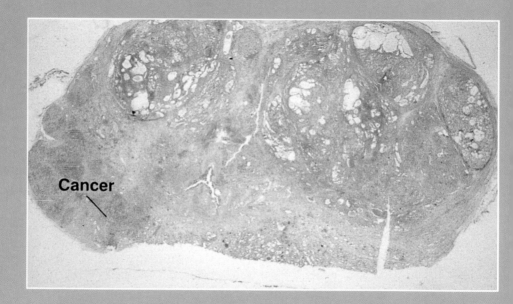

Cancer

Chapter 8

Modern management of prostate cancer

Although prostate cancer is the second most common cause of cancer death in men in most developed countries, there is a surprising lack of consensus concerning its management, especially the treatment of earlier lesions. The principal reason for this is the difficulty in predicting which lesions will progress to the detriment of the patient, as opposed to those which will remain localized and asymptomatic within the affected individual's natural lifespan.

This dilemma is highlighted by the latest statistics on prostate cancer from the USA, which calculate that a man living to 75 years of age has:

- a 30% chance of having microfoci of histological prostate cancer
- a 10% chance of being diagnosed as suffering from clinical disease
- a 2.5% life-time probability of dying from the disease.

Clearly, many men die with prostate cancer rather than as a result of it. However, as the death rate from competing mortalities is falling and the incidence of clinical prostate disease is increasing, the challenge is to identify and effectively treat the life-threatening lesions. In this respect, a shared care approach to the earlier diagnosis and more effective follow-up of prostatic disease between family practitioners and urologists may be beneficial to patients.

Which lesions to treat?

Small-volume microscopic foci of well-differentiated cancer identified at transurethral resection of the prostate (TURP) have little impact on survival and, provided that they are not a harbinger of more significant disease in the peripheral zone, may in older patients often be left untreated[1]. This low-volume, microscopic disease, though present in many men, does not seem to be detectable by current methods of screening.

Larger lesions (> 0.5 cm³) are more dangerous, as are any cancers which are less well-differentiated histologically (Gleason grade > 3)[2]. These tumours are usually, but not always, associated with:

- a serum prostate-specific antigen (PSA) above 4.0 ng/ml
- palpable induration of the prostate (Figure 8.1)
- an abnormal transrectal ultrasound (TRUS) image.

The mortality risk associated with such a lesion must be balanced against the life expectancy of the individual person concerned (i.e. the probability of death from co-morbid conditions, such as cardiovascular disease); clearly the patient's age, general condition and the longevity of his parents will be the dominant considerations.

Management of localized prostate cancers

Unhappily, at present, less than 50% of prostate cancers diagnosed are still confined within the gland. This is probably a reflection of the reluctance of men beyond middle age to consult a doctor about their prostate problems. Those that are detected need to be evaluated by a urologist and carefully staged on the basis of PSA levels, a bone scan, and CT or magnetic resonance imaging (MRI). However, even with the latest endocavity technology, more than 25% of apparently

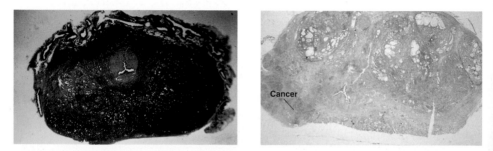

Figure 8.1 *(a) Transverse section of a benign prostate. (b) Localized prostate cancer.*

localized lesions are found to have spread through the prostatic capsule at the time of surgery. For those lesions that are thought to be localized, several treatment options are available.

Watchful waiting

Low-volume lesions. Watchful waiting may be appropriate when the tumour is of low volume and well differentiated, especially in older patients with other significant co-morbid conditions[3]. However, regular review with repeated PSA determination is important in such cases. Active treatment should be considered in younger men if there is evidence of local tumour extension or an incremental PSA rise.

Larger-volume lesions. A more aggressive approach may be appropriate for larger-volume lesions (> 0.5 cm³), containing areas which are less well differentiated, in men with a life expectancy of more than 5–10 years.

Radical radiotherapy

Radical radiotherapy using external beam irradiation has been the mainstay of treatment for localized prostate cancer in much of Europe and to a lesser extent the USA for many years (Figure 8.2). Treatment usually involves two 2-week courses of radiotherapy on an outpatient basis[4]. The morbidity is acceptably low, with the main side-effects being:

- frequency of micturition due to radiation cystitis
- rectal irritation due to the inevitable inclusion of the rectum in the treatment field
- subsequent development of impotence in 30–50% of cases.

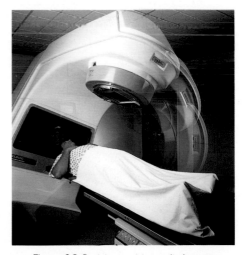

Figure 8.2 *Patient receiving radiotherapy.*

Tumour resistance. Although radiotherapy is well tolerated by both younger and older patients, there is mounting evidence that many prostatic adenocarcinomas – like colonic adenocarcinomas – are relatively resistant to irradiation. Following a period of PSA decline for some months or years after radiotherapy, many patients experience a PSA rise, and this generally heralds a clinical relapse. In addition, several investigators have shown that prostatic biopsies taken 1 year after radiotherapy reveal the presence of viable tumour in 50–60% of patients. Concerns have therefore been raised over the efficacy of radiotherapy in terms of reliable tumour kill; none the less, in older, or less fit, patients with lesions confined to the pelvis, external beam irradiation remains the therapy of choice.

Radical prostatectomy

Radical prostatectomy is the most definitive method of clearing the body of malignant prostate cancer cells if the lesion is still confined within the gland (Figure 8.3 and Table 8.1).

Complications. Concerns about the morbidity associated with the operation have, however, prevented many urologists from using this

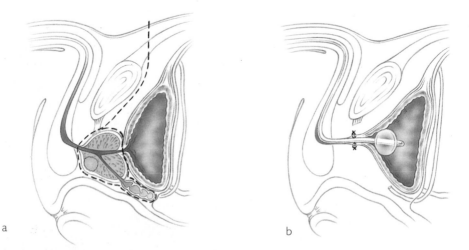

a   b

Figure 8.3 *Radical retropubic prostatectomy. (a) The entire prostate and seminal vesicles are excised. (b) The urethra is anastomosed to the bladder over a 22F catheter which is retained for 2–3 weeks.*

Table 8.1 Comparison of curative therapies for localized prostate cancer

	Invasiveness	Hospital-ization	Complete tumour eradication	Adverse effects
External beam radiotherapy	Nil	Nil	< 50%	Rectal irritation Urinary frequency Impotence (30%)
Radical prosta-tectomy	Retropubic or perineal dissection	6 days	75%	Impotence (50%) Incontinence (2%)

procedure. The recent continence and potency-preserving modifications described and popularized by Dr Patrick Walsh have reduced the complication rates dramatically; many patients remain potent and incontinence – defined as the need for more than two small pads per day – now occurs in less than 2% of cases[5]. Furthermore, the inpatient hospital stay is now only 5–6 days, and the pathological evaluation of the prostate and internal iliac lymph nodes allows precise staging.

Clinical outcome. Providing that the surgical margins are clear, radical prostatectomy reliably reduces serum PSA levels effectively to zero (< 0.5 ng/ml), and this is very helpful during follow-up. Any detectable level of PSA after radical prostatectomy indicates the presence of residual or recurrent tumour, and further adjunctive therapy, usually radiotherapy, should be considered.

The number of radical prostatectomies performed annually under Medicare in the USA has increased from around 8000 to over 32,000 in the last 6 years, and this trend seems likely to be followed elsewhere[6].

Management of locally extensive prostate cancer

A proportion of patients with prostate cancer present with extensive local spread, but no evidence of more distant metastases. For these cancers, radical surgery is probably inappropriate because of the unacceptably high local and distant recurrence rates.

Radiotherapy

Radiotherapy is usually the preferred treatment option, but there is little evidence to suggest that many patients are actually cured by these means, though disease progression may be slowed.

Cytoreduction therapy

Recently, cytoreduction therapy has been in vogue. It comprises a 3-month course of hormonal therapy – usually with a luteinizing hormone releasing hormone (LHRH) analogue, such as goserelin acetate or leuprolide – to achieve tumour shrinkage. Subsequent radiotherapy, or even surgery, may be directed towards a reduced tumour burden. As yet, no controlled studies confirming the enhanced efficacy of this approach over radiotherapy alone have been reported.

Treatment of metastases – androgen blockade

Although the proportion of patients with localized disease at diagnosis is now rising, probably as a result of PSA testing, in many countries more than 50% of patients with prostatic cancer still have metastatic disease at the time of presentation. Since the Nobel prize-winning work of Huggins and Hodges on the hormone dependence of prostate cancer in 1941[7], it has been appreciated that around 70% of such patients will respond to therapy directed towards depriving the cancer cells of the androgens necessary for their growth. This may be accomplished by a variety of means, both medical (Table 8.2) and surgical.

Table 8.2 Medical treatment options for advanced prostate cancer

	Agent	Dose	Side-effects
LHRH analogues	Leuprolide	Monthly	Hot flushes
	Goserelin	(soon	Impotence
	Buserelin	3-monthly)	↓ Libido
Non-steroidal antiandrogens	Flutamide	250 mg t.d.s.	Gynaecomastia
	Nilutamide	300 mg/day	Diarrhoea
	Casodex	150 mg/day	
Progestogenic antiandrogens	Cyproterone acetate	100 mg t.d.s.	Fluid retention Impotence
Oestrogens	Diethyl- stilboestrol	2–5 mg/day	Impotence Gynaecomastia Cardiovascular toxicity

Bilateral orchiectomy

Bilateral orchiectomy can be accomplished in a matter of minutes through a scrotal incision under local, regional or light general anaesthesia, and provides the most cost-effective means of decreasing circulating androgen levels. Although the procedure obviates doctors' worries about compliance, many patients are concerned about the cosmetic and psychological impact of having their testes removed. For this reason, many patients now choose medical means of achieving castration. In a survey performed in 1989, 78% of patients selected medical rather than surgical endocrine therapy for their cancer[8].

LHRH analogues

Shortly after the decapeptide structure of LHRH was elucidated, it was realized that modification of three of the component peptides would result in a compound of greatly increased potency. Chronic administration of these agents results in a temporary increase followed by an inhibition of luteinizing hormone (LH) and follicle stimulating hormone (FSH) release from the pituitary, and a subsequent suppression of testosterone secretion similar to that obtained by surgical castration. At present, three forms of LHRH analogue are available:

- leuprolide
- buserelin
- goserelin acetate.

Leuprolide and goserelin acetate are now available as injectable monthly depot formulations and 3-monthly forms of leuprolide and goserelin are currently under investigation. Buserelin can be administered either intranasally or subcutaneously, but has to be given on a daily basis; a depot preparation is, however, being developed. The depot preparations can be administered in a primary care setting, usually by the practice nurse, in conjunction with less frequent follow-up visits to hospital[9].

On initiation of therapy, all LHRH analogues result in a temporary surge of LH production with a resultant increase in testosterone to 140–170% of basal levels. This effect has been described as the 'flare phenomenon', because of the risk of transient stimulation of prostate tumour growth. This may result in an increase in bone pain and enlargement of spinal metastases with a risk of neurological complications, including paraplegia.

For this reason, it is recommended that for the first 4 weeks after starting an LHRH analogue, adjunctive treatment with an antiandrogen, such as flutamide, 250 mg t.d.s., should be employed.

Prognosis. Although an initial response to androgen deprivation by orchiectomy or LHRH analogue may be obtained in 70–80% of patients, this remission following alteration of the hormonal milieu is not usually maintained in the longer term. The mean time to subsequent tumour progression is less than 18 months, with a mean overall survival time of 18–28 months[9].

Bilateral adrenalectomy

Huggins and Scott[10] were the first to recognize the ephemeral nature of the response of prostate cancer to testicular androgen ablation, and as early as 1945 attempted to treat relapsing patients surgically by bilateral

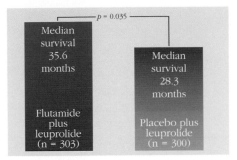

Figure 8.4 *Survival is increased in patients with metastatic cancer given combination therapy with leuprolide and flutamide, compared with those given an LHRH-agonist alone.*

adrenalectomy. Unfortunately, adrenal replacement therapy was less than adequate in these early days and no patient survived longer than 4 months. Nonetheless, this work not only laid the foundation for many future clinical studies of prostatic cancer, but also raised the important question of the contribution of adrenal androgens in sustaining tumour growth once testicular androgens have been withdrawn.

Is monotherapy adequate?

While most urologists have been content to manage patients with advanced prostatic cancer using 'monotherapy' consisting of either bilateral orchiectomy or depot preparations of LHRH analogues, for more than a decade Labrie and co-workers in Canada[11–13] have been urging the therapeutic addition of an antiandrogen to suppress a postulated stimulatory effect by residual androgens of adrenal origin. They have argued that this:

- enhances initial response rates
- delays the development of subsequent androgen independence
- improves both the interval between remission and relapse and overall survival.

However, this approach of 'maximal androgen blockade' has important implications in terms of additional drug toxicity, as well as adding considerably to the economic burden of the disease.

Maximal androgen blockade

Impetus towards a more rigorous evaluation of the clinical effect of maximal androgen blockade came from the demonstration that up to 10–15% of intraprostatic dihydrotestosterone (DHT) remains after medical or surgical castration[14]; moreover, it was confirmed that adrenal androgens may be responsible for as much as 15–20% of total intraprostatic DHT[15].

In response to these observations, a prospective randomized placebo-controlled trial was established in the USA in 1984. The protocol was simple in its design, and compared leuprolide, 1 mg/day subcutaneously, plus placebo with leuprolide, 1 mg/day subcutaneously, plus flutamide, 250 mg t.d.s., in patients with metastatic cancer of the prostate confirmed on radioisotope bone scan. Overall survival was improved in the group receiving flutamide, particularly those with a good performance status and a lesser burden of metastatic disease[16] (Figure 8.4).

Table 8.3 Summary of studies of maximal androgen blockade

Study	Agent	Additional progression-free survival (over monotherapy)	Additional overall survival (over monotherapy)
Crawford et al.[16]	Leuprolide plus flutamide	2.6 months*	7.3 months*
Lungmayr et al.[22]	Goserelin plus flutamide	Nil	Nil
Denis et al.[18]	Goserelin plus flutamide	6 months*	7.3 months*
Janknegt et al.[21]	Orchiectomy plus nilutamide	5.9 months*	7.0 months*

*$p < 0.05$

Other studies comparing various alternative regimens of total androgen blockade with monotherapy have not always revealed such unequivocal advantage[17-23]. None the less, there is a growing consensus about the value of maximum androgen blockade over conventional monotherapy, at least in fitter patients with smaller volumes of metastases (Table 8.3).

Other methods of achieving androgen blockade

Diethylstilboestrol (DES), although inexpensive, is associated with significant cardiovascular toxicity at doses of 5 mg/day or 3 mg/day. This toxicity is reduced at a dose of 1 mg/day, but serum testosterone levels are not reliably suppressed into the castrate range[24]. One European study, however, in which patients were randomized to either DES, 1 mg/day, or bilateral orchiectomy, with or without cyproterone acetate, showed no differences in either survival or cardiovascular thromboembolic events. DES also causes troublesome gynaecomastia (Figure 8.5) and, in most circumstances, is no longer first-line therapy for prostate cancer.

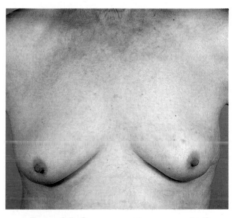

Figure 8.5 *Gynaecomastia as a result of diethylstilboestrol therapy.*

Cyproterone acetate and megestrol acetate are steroidal antiandrogens, both of which have marked progestational activity, which inhibits LH release from the pituitary and produces castrate levels of testosterone; they also compete with testosterone and dihydrotestosterone (DHT) for androgen receptor sites. However, if either cyproterone acetate or megestrol acetate is used as monotherapy, there tends to be a gradual increase in testosterone values with chronic usage as a result of gradual loss of pituitary inhibition, and these agents are probably not as effective as DES or orchiectomy. Few data demonstrating their value in combination with LHRH analogues or orchiectomy are yet available, but a similar benefit to that seen with the non-steroidal antiandrogens, flutamide and nilutamide might be anticipated.

Cyproterone acetate, in doses as low as 50 mg/day, is also useful in the treatment of the troublesome 'hot flushes' that may result from androgen withdrawal following orchiectomy or LHRH analogue therapy.

Flutamide is a non-steroidal antiandrogen which has been used as monotherapy for metastatic prostate cancer. It has not, however, received regulatory approval for this indication and, at present, flutamide should always be used in conjunction with either medical or surgical castration. There are data to suggest that, when flutamide is used as monotherapy, it leaves 40% of androgen receptor sites still available for binding by DHT; when combined with castration, however, only 5% of DHT is able to interact with androgen receptors.

Unlike most other agents active against prostate cancer, flutamide when used alone does not usually affect libido and potency. Diarrhoea however is not uncommon, and gynaecomastia and breast tenderness also occur, presumably because of increased aromatization of testosterone to oestradiol. These latter effects are not seen when flutamide is combined with an LHRH analogue, such as leuprolide, goserelin or buserelin.

Nilutamide is another non-steroidal antiandrogen similar to flutamide. In contrast to cyproterone acetate, nilutamide is devoid of progestational and antigonadotrophic properties. It competes with testosterone and DHT at the androgen receptor, not only at the level of the prostate, but also at the hypothalamo-pituitary complex (where androgens exert their negative feedback effect). As a result, LH secretion is enhanced and, in the presence of intact testes, testosterone biosynthesis is increased. However, because of the presence of the antiandrogen, the effects of the rising testosterone at the receptor level are blunted. Theoretically therefore nilutamide, like flutamide, is not ideal as monotherapy and there are currently no data to support its use in this context. Its main value seems to be in combination with an LHRH analogue. Side-effects of nilutamide include gastrointestinal symptoms, anaemia and disturbances of light/dark adaptation.

Casodex (ICI 176334) is a new non-steroidal antiandrogen that binds to the androgen receptor in the rat prostate with about 2% of the affinity of DHT, but roughly four times the affinity of flutamide. Unlike flutamide, Casodex does not cause a marked elevation in serum LH and testosterone in rats or dogs, and has a long half-life[25]. Phase II clinical trials revealed reasonable efficacy of Casodex, 50 mg/day, when used as monotherapy in patients with metastatic prostate cancer, as judged by both serum acid phosphatase and PSA level decline. The most common side-effects were breast tenderness, gynaecomastia and hot flushes; however, the incidence of hot flushes was lower in those receiving Casodex (19%) than those treated by orchiectomy (58%). In contrast to the preclinical animal studies, in man, Casodex does, like flutamide, appear to elevate serum testosterone levels markedly, due to central antagonism of T receptors in the hypothalamo pituitary complex with a consequent increase in LH secretion[26]. This has led to concern about its ability to block androgen receptors completely in the nuclei of androgen-sensitive cells. However, Casodex has a long half-life which enables high serum concentrations to be maintained; moreover, in patients treated with Casodex, serum testosterone concentrations rarely exceed the normal levels at the androgen receptor that the drug must antagonize.

Phase III studies are currently under way comparing Casodex, 150 mg/day, as monotherapy with either the LHRH analogue, goserelin, or orchiectomy. Its low toxicity profile and once-daily dose regimen makes it a strong candidate for the future – either as monotherapy or in combination with an LHRH analogue – for patients with prostate cancer.

Finasteride is a 4-azasteroid competitor of 5-alpha reductase 2, the enzyme that converts testosterone to DHT within the prostate, which is also used as therapy for BPH. Several studies have confirmed that finasteride reduces serum DHT by 60–75% while maintaining testosterone levels, and results in significant regression of the benignly enlarged gland[27]. Finasteride has been associated with a marked decline in intraprostatic DHT, but a rise in intraprostatic testosterone levels. Animal studies have suggested that finasteride would have activity in prostate cancer[28], and a pilot study in 28 patients with metastatic prostate cancer showed a small reduction in PSA, rather less than that seen after orchiectomy or treatment with an LHRH analogue[29]. It seems likely that androgen receptors in prostate cancer metastases do not demonstrate the selective responsiveness to DHT, as opposed to testosterone, that characterizes both normal prostate and BPH tissue. However, a study of 120 patients randomized to either finasteride or placebo after radical prostatectomy showed an 18-month delay in PSA rise in the drug treatment group[30]. Finasteride in combination with an antiandrogen might also have some efficacy without inducing impotence.

Finasteride is a competitive inhibitor of 5-alpha reductase, while other inhibitors, such as the new agent episteride (SK&F 105657), are uncompetitive inhibitors. A recent report of the use of episteride in androgen-responsive cell lines and in R-3327 tumour-bearing rats suggested some potentially useful anti-tumour activity[31]. However, the results of phase II trials into the effect of this compound in patients have not yet been reported. The appeal of a 5-alpha-reductase inhibitor in this context is the very favourable toxicity profile compared with the other agents discussed above; virtually the only side-effect seen with finasteride is a 3–5% incidence of impotence, which is reversible on discontinuation of the drug.

Timing of endocrine ablation for metastatic prostate cancer

Traditionally, urologists have favoured deferred administration of hormonal manipulation in patients with prostate cancer – often waiting until symptoms appear before acting to ablate testicular androgens. The rationale for this decision to delay therapy was largely based on a study that showed no difference in average survival rates between patients given hormonal therapy, and those in whom hormonal therapy was withheld and placebo given until they became symptomatic[32]. However, recent re-analysis of these data, in which deaths due to cardiovascular events in the oestrogen-treated group were excluded and cancer-specific death rates were calculated, showed that patients who were treated initially with oestrogen therapy fared better than those treated with placebo[33].

It is now generally agreed that prompt intervention in patients who present with metastatic disease is beneficial, both in terms of time to progression and overall survival.

Management of 'hormone-escaped' metastatic prostate cancer

Unfortunately almost all prostate cancers after a period of response to androgen ablation eventually begin to grow again; this is termed 'hormone escape'. Ideally, second-line therapy to obtain a second remission would be used, as in the management of carcinoma of the breast. Unfortunately, no second-line therapy has confirmed efficacy in this respect, though a number of agents, including Estramustine, mitomycin C, epirubicin, liarozole[34] and the growth factor inhibitor Suramin, are currently being tested in this context. Prednisolone in high doses may also produce a useful symptomatic response, though the mechanism is still unclear.

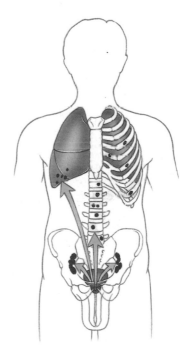

The most common clinical problem is debilitating bone pain from bone metastases (Figure 8.6). Local radiotherapy to painful areas may be also of value or, if the discomfort and deposits are very diffuse, intravenous strontium-89[35] may achieve useful palliation.

Figure 8.6 *Prostatic cancer commonly spreads to lymph nodes, bones and lungs.*

However, despite all efforts, most patients with hormone-escaped prostate cancer deteriorate remorselessly and die within a few months of the first signs of relapse.

Looking ahead

The optimal management of prostate cancer now requires care to be shared between the urologist and the family practitioner. The initial treatment strategy should be devised by a specialist on the basis of a tissue diagnosis and careful staging. Radical radiotherapy or total prostatectomy are obviously the province of the hospital-based team, but follow-up can be the joint responsibility of urologist and family practitioner. Metastatic disease is increasingly managed by monthly depot injections of LHRH analogues and these may, in some circumstances, be administered by the family practitioner rather than the urologist. The family practitioner may also play a key role in the palliative therapy and terminal care of patients with advanced disease.

The hypothesis that androgen precursors secreted by the adrenal glands may play a role in maintaining prostate cancer growth and the escape of tumour cells from hormone control after ablation of testicular androgens is gaining credence. There is strong evidence that a subgroup of patients with 'good performance' (i.e. those that are in good general condition) and a reasonably restricted volume of metastatic disease may, in fact, remain in remission longer and have a more prolonged survival if treated by total androgen blockade, as opposed to conventional monotherapy.

In the future, it may be possible to predict, by biochemical or morphometric means, a subgroup of patients in whom total androgen blockade, rather than monotherapy, may offer a definite survival advantage. Newer, more effective first- and second-line therapies also need to be developed. These challenges may be added to the many others that must be overcome in order to reduce the morbidity and mortality of this most prevalent disease.

Summary

■ Optimal management of prostate cancer requires shared care between urologists and family practitioners.

■ Microscopic foci of well-differentiated prostate cancer have little impact on survival and often require no treatment, especially in older men, while larger lesions (> 0.5 cm³) and those which are moderately or poorly differentiated carry a poorer prognosis and may warrant more aggressive treatment.

■ Curative treatment options for prostate cancer include radical prostatectomy and external beam radiotherapy. Locally advanced lesions may be treated by prior hormonal manipulation (cytoreduction) followed by external beam radiotherapy.

■ Metastatic prostate cancer is usually treated by androgen withdrawal, which has a response rate of about 70%. Treatment options include bilateral orchiectomy or the use of LHRH analogues. The use of oestrogens is associated with an increased risk of cardiovascular side-effects and gynaecomastia.

■ The addition of an antiandrogen, such as flutamide or nilutamide, to achieve 'maximal androgen blockade' by neutralizing the 5% of residual androgens secreted from the adrenal glands, may increase both the time to disease progression and provide a survival advantage in some patients with less advanced metastatic disease.

■ Current second-line therapies after relapse are usually ineffectual.

■ Palliative treatment, which is often the province of the family practitioner, is usually given for bone pain or anaemia. It involves the use of blood transfusions, steroids, local radiotherapy and intravenous strontium-89, but seldom significantly improves survival.

References

1 Matzkin H, Patel JP, Altwein JE, Soloway MS. Stage T1A carcinoma of the prostate. *Urology* 1994; **43**: 11–21.

2 McNeal JE, Bostwick DG, Kindrachuk RA, Redwine EA, Freiha FS, Stamey TA. Patterns of progression in prostate cancer. *Lancet* 1986; **i**: 60–3.

3 George NJR. Natural history of localized prostate cancer managed by conservative therapy above. *Lancet* 1988; **i**: 494–7.

4 Bagshaw MA, Cox RS, Ramback JE. Radiation therapy for localized prostate cancer. *Int J Radiol Biol Phys* 1986; **12**: 1721–7.

5 Catalona WJ, Bigg SW. Nerve-sparing radical prostatectomy: evaluation of results after 250 patients. *J Urol* 1990; **143**: 538–44.

6 Lu-Yao GL, Greenburg ER. Changes in prostate cancer incidence and treatment in the USA. *Lancet* 1994; **343**: 251-4.

7 Huggins C, Hodges CV. Studies of prostatic cancer: I Effect of castration, oestrogen and androgen injections on serum phosphates in metastatic carcinoma of the prostate. *Canc Res* 1941; **1**: 293–7.

8 Cassileth BR. Patients' choice of treatment in stage D prostate cancer. *Urology* 1989; **33 (suppl 5)**: 57–61.

9 Debruyne FMJ. Long-term therapy with a depot luteinizing hormone-releasing hormone analogue (Zoladex) in patients with advanced prostatic carcinoma. *J Urol* 1988; **140**: 775–7.

10 Huggins C, Scott WW. Bilateral adrenalectomy in prostate cancer. *Ann Surg* 1945; **122**: 1031-41.

11 Labrie F, Dupont A, Giguere AU. Combination therapy with flutamide and castration (orchidectomy or LHRH agonists) the minimal therapy in both treated and previously treated patients. *J Steroid Biochem* 1987; **27**: 525–32.

12 Labrie F. Benefits of combination therapy with flutamide in patients relapsing after castration. *Br J Urol* 1988; **61**: 341.

13 Labrie F, Dupont A, Belanger A. Combination therapy with flutamide and castration (LHRH agonist or orchidectomy) in advanced prostate cancer: a marked improvement in response and survival. *J Steroid Biochem* 1985; **23**: 833–41.

14 Geller J, De La Vega DJ, Albert JD. Tissue dihydrotestosterone levels and clinical response to hormone therapy in patients with prostate cancer. *J Clin Endocrinol Metab* 1984; **58**: 36–40.

15 Harper ME, Pike A, Peeling WB. Steroids of adrenal origin metabolized by human prostate tissue both in vivo and in vitro. *J Endocrinol* 1984; **60**: 117.

16 Crawford ED, Eisenberger MA, McLeod DG *et al*. A controlled trial of leuprolide with and without flutamide in prostatic cancer. *N Engl J Med* 1989; **321**: 419–24.

17 Mayer FJ, Crawford ED. Optimal therapy for metastatic prostate cancer. In: Hendry WF, Kirby RS, eds. *Recent advances in urology/andrology*. Edinburgh: Churchill Livingstone, 1994: 159–75.

18 Denis LJ. Treatment of M1 prostatic cancer: update of the EORTC trials. Special report plenary session 1. *American Urological Association Scientific Meeting, 1992.* Washington DC.

19 Keuppens F, Denis L, Smith P. Zoladex and flutamide versus bilateral orchidectomy. A randomized phase III EORTC 30853 study. *Cancer* 1990; **66**: 1045–57.

20 Canadian Anandron Study Group. Total androgen blockade in the treatment of metastatic prostate cancer. *Seminar Urol* 1990; **8**: 159.

21 Janknegt RA. International Anandron Study Group: Efficacy and tolerance of a total androgen blockade with Anandron and orchidectomy. A double-blind, placebo controlled multicentre study. *J Urol* 1991; **145**: 425A.

22 Lungmayr A. The international prostate cancer study group. A multicentre trial comparing the LHRH analogue Zoladex, with Zoladex plus flutamide in the treatment of advanced prostate cancer. *Eur Urol* 1990; **18 (suppl 3)**: 28–9.

23 Iversen P, Sucini S, Sylvester R. Zoladex and flutamide versus orchidectomy in the treatment of advanced prostate cancer. A combined analysis of two European studies EORTC and DAPROCA 86. *Cancer* 1990, **66**: 1067–73.

24 Shearer RJ, Hendry WF, Sommerville IF. Plasma testosterone, an accurate monitor of hormone treatment in prostate cancer. *Br J Urol* 1973; **45**: 668.

25 Furr BJA, Valcaccia B, Curry B. ICI 1/6334. A novel non-steroidal peripherally selective antiandrogen. *J Endocrinol* 1987; **113**: R7-R9.

26 Kennealey GT, Furr BJA. Use of the non-steroidal antiandrogen Casodex in advanced prostatic cancer. *Urol Clin North America* 1991; **18**: 99–110.

27 Gormley GJ, Stoner E, Bruskewitz RC *et al.* The effect of finasteride in men with benign prostatic hyperplasia. *N Engl J Med* 1992; **327**: 1185–91.

28 Brooks JR, Berman C, Nguyen H *et al.* Effect of castration, DES, flutamide, and the 5-alpha reductase inhibitor MK906, on the growth of the Dunning rat prostatic carcinoma, R-3327. *Prostate* 1991; **18**: 215–17.

29 Presti JC, Fair WC, Andriole G. Multicentre randomised double-blind, placebo controlled study to investigate the effect of finasteride (MK906) on stage D prostate cancer. *J Urol* 1992; **148**: 1201–4.

30 Andriole G, Block N, Boake R. Two years of treatment with finasteride after radical prostatectomy. *J Urol* 1994; **151**: 435A.

31 Lamb JC, Levy MA, Johnson RK, Issacs JT. Response of rat and human prostatic tumours to the novel 5-alpha reductase inhibitor, SK&F 105657. *Prostate* 1992; **21**: 15–34.

32 Veterans Administration Cooperative Urological Research Group. Carcinoma of the prostate: treatment comparisons. *J Urol* 1967; **98**: 516–19.

33 Sarosdy MF. Do we have a national treatment plan for stage D1 carcinoma of the prostate? *World J Urol* 1990; **8**: 27–32.

34 Dijkman GA, Mooreselaam RJ, Finckel RV. Antitumoral effects of liarozole in androgen dependent and undependent, R–3327 running prostate adenocarcinomas. *J Urol* 1994; **151**: 217–22.

35 Laing AH, Ackery DM, Bayly RJ *et al.* Strontium-89 chloride for pain palliation in prostatic skeletal malignancy. *Br J Radiol* 1991; **64**: 816–822.

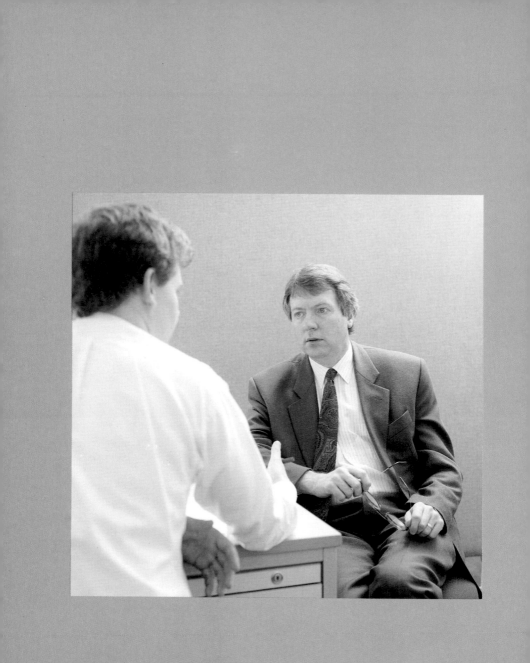

Chapter 9

Shared care in practice: case studies

Case 1: Severe prostatism

A 67-year-old man presents to his family practitioner with frequency, nocturia and poor stream. The only abnormal physical sign is marked enlargement of the prostate on digital rectal examination (DRE). How would you proceed?

Family practitioner. Start by taking a careful history, enquiring about nocturia, strength of stream and the degree of bother that the symptoms cause – the so-called 'three questions' (Table 5.2). Then ask the patient to complete an International Prostate Symptom Score (IPSS) sheet (Table 5.4). The impact of the problem on the individual's quality of life is an important consideration. Perform a careful DRE, and send blood for urea and electrolytes (U&E), full blood count (FBC) and prostate-specific antigen (PSA) determination. Also arrange for dipstick testing and if positive an MSU. If the symptoms were sufficiently bothersome to the patient for treatment to be considered, refer him for a bladder ultrasound to determine the post-void residual (PVR) volume and a uroflow determination.

Results

Three questions	All positive
IPSS	21
FBC	Normal
U&E	Normal
Serum creatinine	Normal
PSA	5.8 ng/ml
MSU	Negative
Bladder ultrasound	BPH, PVR 350 ml
Maximum flow rate	6.1 ml/second

Family practitioner. This patient has severe prostatic symptoms which bother him. His PSA is mildly elevated, but this is probably consistent with the palpable degree of prostatic enlargement. The results show a significant PVR and a markedly reduced flow rate with

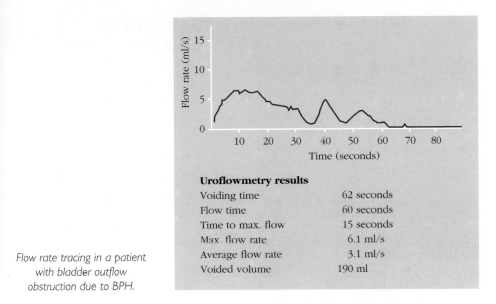

Uroflowmetry results

Voiding time	62 seconds
Flow time	60 seconds
Time to max. flow	15 seconds
Max. flow rate	6.1 ml/s
Average flow rate	3.1 ml/s
Voided volume	190 ml

Flow rate tracing in a patient with bladder outflow obstruction due to BPH.

an abnormal IPSS. These findings suggest the need for surgery, and the patient should be referred to a urologist.

Urologist. This patient should be referred for urological evaluation, but remember not all men with palpably enlarged prostates are obstructed. There are several danger signs associated with this case. The severity of the symptoms associated with considerable obstruction suggest that pharmacotherapy is unlikely to be sufficient. Moreover, the mildly raised PSA, while probably the result of BPH, requires careful assessment because of the 20% or so probability of prostate cancer. A urologist would re-examine the prostate and recheck the PSA.

This patient requires a TURP. The only issue that the purists would debate is whether pressure-flow studies are required in order to document absolutely the presence of obstruction. The patient has presented with symptoms of obstruction for which he seeks treatment. He has a very low flow rate with a very high PVR. Even taking into account the risk *versus* benefit ratio (or balance-sheet concept), surgical treatment should be instituted, with a high expectation of symptom resolution.

Case 2: Post-micturition dribble

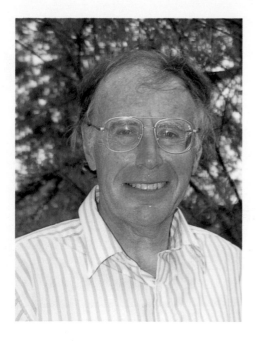

A 56-year-old man presents with post-micturition dribble, but a reportedly normal flow rate. His prostate felt normal on DRE. How would you proceed?

Family practitioner. Patients with this fairly common presentation have little in the way of significant pathology, but are basically seeking reassurance. Referral to a urologist is inappropriate, unless the patient requires further reassurance. The answers to the 'three questions' are usually all negative and the IPSS is less than 8. Counsel the patient about post-micturition dribble, informing him that it is a common and benign symptom due to pooling of urine in the bulbar urethra. Also measure PSA to establish a baseline and ask for an MSU to exclude microscopic haematuria or urinary tract infection (UTI).

Urologist. Post-micturition dribble is usually the result of pooling of urine in the bulbar urethra after the distal urethral sphincter has closed. Normally the bulbo-cavernosus muscles – which are the ejaculatory muscles – contract around the urethra to expel the last few drops of urine. With time, however, and particularly after any kind of urethral surgery, they function less well with the result that post-micturition dribble occurs. No invasive therapy is indicated. The individual should be advised to exert pressure in the perineum immediately after micturition to empty the bulbar urethra into the

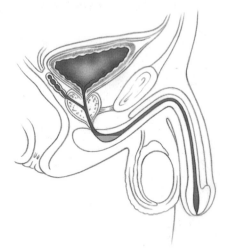

After micturition, a few millilitres of urine pools in the bulbar urethra. Pressure in the perineum massages urine into the pendulous urethra and resolves the problem.

pendulous urethra from which it will drain by gravity. Referral is unnecessary in these patients.

Occasionally patients with urethral strictures, or a 'baggy' urethra due to previous surgery for stricture disease, may present with these symptoms, in which case a urethrogram may be indicated. Patients with strictures usually admit to a very poor stream and the flow rate is markedly reduced.

Case 3: Asymptomatic, concerned patient

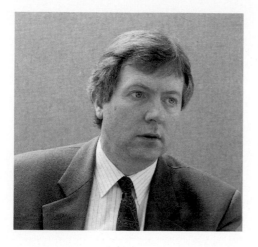

A 50-year-old man attends the family practice requesting a prostate health check having read about prostate problems in a newspaper. How would you proceed?

Family practitioner. First ascertain whether this man has, in fact, any urinary symptoms by asking the 'three questions'. Then ask him to complete the IPSS score. It is also advisable to assess his level of knowledge, worries and expectations. Perform a DRE, which would probably be normal in this case, run through some routine laboratory investigations including serum creatinine and PSA, and send urine off for culture and microscopy.

Results

Three questions	All negative
IPSS	5
DRE	Normal
Serum creatinine	Normal
PSA	1.6 ng/ml
MSU	Normal

Family practitioner. All these results are normal. The patient is effectively asymptomatic and he is really looking for reassurance about prostate cancer. With a PSA value of 1.6 ng/ml, advise him that the chances of prostate cancer are extremely low and that no action is necessary, but he should return to the clinic in 1 year's time for a repeat DRE and PSA determination.

Encouraging the adoption of a more healthy life-style, including a balanced diet may be beneficial for the patient.

Urologist. It is worth asking the patient whether or not there are any first-degree relatives who developed carcinoma of the prostate, particularly at a young age. There is certainly nothing to suggest either outflow obstruction or prostate cancer, and no indication for referring him for ultrasound studies, flowometry or transrectal ultrasonography, but a repeat PSA after 1 year is advisable in a man with these sorts of anxieties. A PSA increment of more than 20% (or > 0.75 ng/ml) over 1 year can be an indication of developing localized prostate cancer. In a recent study from Seattle, USA, 17% of patients whose PSA levels were originally less than 4 ng/ml, but which rose by more than 20% over 1 year, were found to have prostate cancer when sextant transrectal prostate biopsies were performed.

Case 4: Fever, frequency, dysuria

A man aged 45 presents with a fever, frequency and dysuria of 10 days' duration. On examination, he has an enlarged and rather 'boggy'-feeling prostate, which is acutely tender on examination. How would you manage this individual?

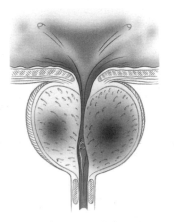

In patients with acute prostatitis, the prostate will feel 'boggy' and be acutely tender.

Family practitioner. This kind of history and physical findings suggests a diagnosis of UTI with acute prostatitis. Send the urine specimen for culture, check his serum PSA and serum creatinine together with an FBC and ESR, and start this patient on an aminoquinolone antibiotic. Then arrange to see him in 1 week's time when the results of these investigations would be available. If there has been no response to treatment by then, consider a referral.

Results

MSU	WBC +++, *Escherichia coli* on culture
Serum creatinine	Normal
FBC	WBC 15.5
PSA	40 ng/ml

Family practitioner. These results suggest acute prostatitis. The patient will most likely respond to antibiotics, so plan to keep him on this medication for at least another 3 weeks. Send another MSU at 1 week to see whether the culture at this stage is negative and whether there is any change in the sensitivities of the organism. Allow at least 3 months to lapse before repeating the PSA, which should then have fallen quite steeply. It would also be advisable to image the kidneys by ultrasound.

Symptoms of acute bacterial prostatitis

- Fever/malaise
- Pain on ejaculation
- Perineal, low back and rectal pain
- Urinary urgency and frequency
- Nocturia and dysuria
- Bladder neck obstruction of varying degrees

Urologist. This case certainly is suggestive of a UTI with associated acute prostatitis. The only concern about these patients is that they can occasionally develop an intraprostatic abscess and, in these situations, oral antibiotics may not always penetrate the abscess and sterilize the lesion. Occasionally, the patient needs to be hospitalized and the abscess drained surgically. In addition, patients with acute prostatitis can develop quite severe symptoms of bladder outflow obstruction and occasionally even develop acute urinary retention.

An elevated PSA of 40 ng/ml is not at all surprising in a case like this, and is an indication of the degree of disruption to the prostate caused by the acute infection. As mentioned above, the PSA would be expected to drop to normal values within 3 months or so of therapy. If this did not occur, then the patient should be referred for biopsy to exclude any coincidental malignant process within the prostate.

Case 5: Moderate prostatism and hard nodule

A man aged 62 presents with moderate symptoms of prostatism of at least 2 years' duration. On examination, however, his prostate is not enlarged, but has a small nodule about 1.5 cm in diameter, which is palpable in the left lobe of the prostate. What are the next steps?

Family practitioner. Clearly, both some degree of BPH and concomitant prostate cancer would be suspected in this patient. Check FBC, U&E and creatinine, and send blood for PSA level determination. Refer him urgently, there and then, to a urologist and chase up the PSA results.

Results

FBC	Normal
U&E/serum creatinine	Normal
MSU	Negative
PSA	12.5 ng/ml

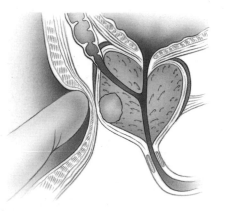

Small palpable nodule on the left lobe of the prostate.

Family practitioner. This PSA result in the absence of much prostatic enlargement and in the presence of a palpable nodule, strongly suggests the presence of prostate cancer. In a man of this age, his evaluation by a urologist should be expedited.

Urologist. A man with a PSA of 12.5 ng/ml and a nodule in the prostate has a more than 60% chance of having prostate cancer on biopsy. He needs a transrectal ultrasound (TRUS)-guided biopsy of the nodule on the left side, as well as random quadrant or preferably sextant biopsies through the rest of the prostate to determine whether or not other concomitant foci of cancer are present.

Results

Biopsy	Gleason grade 4, well-differentiated cancer in two of the biopsies from the left lobe. All the other biopsies revealed benign tissue

Urologist. These findings suggest the presence of significant volume cancer in one lobe of the prostate. Provided that the patient had no other significant cardiovascular or respiratory disease, we would want to stage the disease by taking an MRI scan of the prostate and pelvic lymph nodes, together with a bone scan to exclude the presence of either lymphatic metastases in the internal iliac lymph nodes or, more commonly, bone metastases. A recent study found that more than half the patients with a PSA greater than 10 ng/ml had cancer which was beyond the confines of the prostatic capsule.

Results

Bone scan	Negative
MRI scan	No evidence of extracapsular seminal vesicle or internal iliac lymph node involvement by tumour

Urologist. The treatment options in this patient are radical radiotherapy *versus* radical prostatectomy. Unfortunately, there is no adequately conducted head-to-head randomized prospective study of these modalities of treatment to guide us, but many urologists now believe that radical prostatectomy is more effective in younger patients with organ-confined lesions than radiotherapy. This is because radiotherapy does not reliably bring down the PSA to undetectable levels or render the patient tumour free on repeat transrectal biopsy at 1 year in more than 50% of cases. A new treatment modality, cryosurgery to the prostate, is currently being evaluated in the USA, but at this stage must be considered investigational.

A patient in his early 60s with a biopsy-proven carcinomatous prostatic nodule (stage T2a or T2b) should probably have a radical prostatectomy or radical radiotherapy if his bone scan is negative. With surgery, the patient is usually discharged from hospital after 7 days, with the urethral catheter *in situ*. He is readmitted to the day ward 2 weeks later for removal of the catheter. There may be some initial frequency and urgency, but this usually clears up quickly. There may also be some early stress incontinence, but in an otherwise healthy 62-year-old man, this should not persist. In older patients, stress incontinence may be present for a somewhat longer period of time, but urinary continence is regained eventually in most patients. Erectile impotence may occur despite the use of a nerve-sparing technique; however, most patients respond to self-injection therapy with papaverine or prostaglandin E1.

This individual did undergo a radical retropubic prostatectomy that confirmed that the tumour, which contained areas of Gleason grade 6 adenocarcinoma, was confined to the left lobe of the prostate which extended up to, but did not obviously involve, the capsule on the left-hand side. Postoperatively, he did well with no stress incontinence after removal of his catheter. His PSA remains below 0.5 ng/ml at the time of writing.

Case 6: Prostatism, low back pain

A 65-year-old man presents with a history of low back pain with concomitant symptoms of prostatism. Clinical examination reveals some tenderness of the lumbar spine with restricted movements, and DRE reveals an irregular stony hard prostate. What are the next steps in this situation?

Family practitioner. The clear suspicion here is prostatic cancer with skeletal metastases, so proceed with the initial investigations of a FBC, U&E and serum creatinine together with a PSA determination, radiographs of the lumbar spine and a request for a bone scan. Urgently refer the patient to a urologist.

Results

FBC	Normal
U&E	Normal
Serum creatinine	Normal
PSA	249 ng/ml
X-rays	Lumbar spine – evidence of sclerotic deposits in the lumbar spine and pelvis
Bone scan	Positive for multiple metastases
TRUS	Hypo-echoic areas suggestive of prostate cancer and capsular distortion
Biopsy	Positive for adenocarcinoma Gleason grade 9

Urologist. This is a classical case of a patient with metastatic prostate carcinoma. Unfortunately, more than 50% of patients currently presenting with prostate cancer are found to have either locally extensive or metastatic disease, and curative therapy in such cases is not possible. A patient like this would certainly be best treated with hormone therapy and at present there is evidence to suggest that the combination of either orchiectomy or the use of a luteinizing hormone

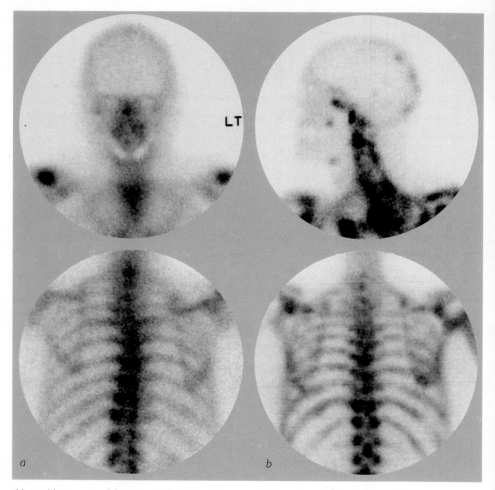

Normal bone scans (a) contrasted with positive scans (b) showing multiple 'hot spots' due to metastatic prostate cancer. This patient's PSA was 430 ng/ml.

releasing hormone (LHRH) analogue plus an antiandrogen, usually flutamide, 250 mg t.d.s., or cyproterone acetate, 100 mg t.d.s. The rationale behind the addition of these antiandrogens to either orchiectomy or the LHRH analogue is to block the effect of the 5% or so of androgens still circulating, which are secreted by the adrenal glands. In such circumstances, about 70% of men would be expected

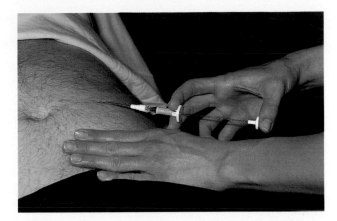

Injection of depot LHRH analogue as treatment for metastatic prostate cancer.

to respond with a rapid PSA decline. There would also be a rapid improvement in the patient's symptoms. Hormone manipulation, as described above, gives the most effective pain relief, and, in many cases, no further analgesia is required. Unfortunately, a long-term response to treatment cannot be guaranteed: about half the patients will suffer PSA relapse within 18–24 months and there is a 50% mortality within 36 months.

Follow-up and palliative control of metastatic bone pain is very much in the province of the family practitioner – ideally in consultation and collaboration with the urologist.

Case 7: Bothersome prostatism, reluctance to undergo surgery

A 56-year-old man presents with bothersome urinary symptoms. On examination his prostate gland is enlarged, but feels benign, and his PSA level is at the upper limit of normal at 3.9 ng/ml. The patient has recently remarried and has read about medical therapy in the press and is keen to avoid any kind of surgical intervention. How do you manage this problem?

Family practitioner. This patient seems to have obstructive BPH, so his answers to the 'three questions' will probably be positive and his IPSS can be expected to be above normal. Check that his prostate is only benignly enlarged on DRE and that his PSA is within normal limits. Before starting medical therapy and if possible, obtain a flow rate and then ultrasound determination of PVR. At present, both ultrasound and flow rate measurements are obtained through the local hospital, the report coming back to the practice.

Results	
IPSS	14
PSA	3.9 ng/ml
Maximum flow rate	9.6 ml/second
PVR	120 ml

Family practitioner. These results are consistent with bladder outflow obstruction due to BPH, and medical treatment is appropriate. His PSA is, however, at the upper limit of normal, and it would be advisable to discuss this with a urologist over the telephone. The current choice of medical treatments is between the 5-alpha-reductase inhibitor finasteride, or one of the newer longer-acting alpha blockers. As the symptom relief afforded by the 5-alpha-reductase inhibitor can take several months to become evident, a combination of both finasteride and an alpha blocker, such as terazosin, starting off at 2 mg/day and gradually titrating to 5 mg/day over a month, could be used.

Before patients are started on alpha blockers, they should be warned that about 10% of patients may experience drowsiness or mild dizziness, and occasionally nasal stuffiness. Finasteride has a very good side-effect profile, though about 3–5% of patients will experience reduced libido and occasionally impotence.

Follow-up of patients on medical therapy for BPH is important, and they should be assessed at 3-monthly intervals. After 1 year of therapy, repeat the ultrasound and flow rate measurements, and request a new PSA which would be expected to have fallen to around 50% of the pre-treatment value as a result of the effect of finasteride on the PSA-elaborating epithelium. If the subjective and objective response is good, continue therapy indefinitely.

Urologist. It is certainly unnecessary these days for every patient of this type to be referred to a urologist, but it does mean that the family practitioner will have to move up the learning curve in terms of the interpretation of flow rate measurements, PVR determinations and PSA results. Discussion with a urologist will be useful if any doubt exists. As has been mentioned above, the use of finasteride would be expected to result in significant reduction of PSA; the median decline in those patients treated in the phase III double-blind studies was 50%. Those patients with carcinoma of the prostate who were inadvertently included in the phase III studies showed a much smaller decline in PSA and, in most cases, after an initial decline, the PSA value started to rise. These findings indicate that those patients in whom the PSA level does not fall significantly, and especially those in whom a PSA rise is seen in spite of therapy compliance with finasteride, 5 mg/day, should be referred for TRUS and prostatic biopsy to exclude prostate cancer. Patients need to be educated about the continued need for compliance, as the beneficial effects of finasteride take time to develop. At present, however, compliance does not seem to be a problem.

Case 8: Acute urinary retention, sexual concerns

A 58-year-old man who has a much younger wife and has been known to have prostatic symptoms for some time, but who has been managed by watchful waiting because of worries about sexual dysfunction resulting from surgery, has recently presented to the local Accident and Emergency Department with acute urinary retention. A catheter was passed and he was told that surgery is likely to be necessary, but this will almost inevitably induce retrograde ejaculation. He was discharged home with his catheter *in situ,* and subsequently presents to the family practitioner to discuss the possibilities of alternatives to surgery in the management of his urinary retention.

Family practitioner. Refer this patient to a urologist. Medical treatment with 5-alpha-reductase inhibitors or alpha blockers are not of any great value once outflow obstruction has reached the stage of acute urinary retention. While he is in the surgery, however, perform a DRE, and take blood for a PSA determination and a specimen of urine from the catheter for microscopy and culture.

Results

DRE	Marked BPH
Microscopy	RBC +++
Urine culture	Negative
PSA	9.3 ng/ml

Urologist. In patients who present with acute retention of urine, the only recognized management at present is transurethral resection of the prostate (TURP) or open prostatectomy. The results of this form of treatment are excellent, with the virtual assurance for the patient of a satisfactory outcome.

We are seeing quite a few patients now who have acute urinary retention, but are *determined* to avoid TURP and are requesting alternative forms of therapy. Unfortunately, none of the new non-surgical forms of intervention can reliably re-establish voiding in these cases. Balloon dilatation is usually unsuccessful. Hyperthermia or thermotherapy using the Prostatron device also has an unacceptably high failure rate, and prostatic stents are used only in a highly-selected group of patients, particularly those

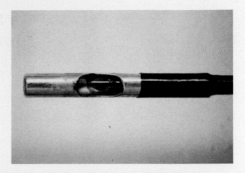

Side-firing laser prostatectomy probe.

with severe, concurrent illness. Other than a standard TURP, the only treatment that could be considered at present is a laser-assisted prostatectomy. Before undertaking endoscopic laser ablation of the prostate (ELAP), however, the patient must understand clearly that this is a new technique that should, at this stage, be regarded as investigational. With the use of a side-firing laser fibre, we have managed to re-establish voiding in several patients such as those who are very keen to avoid the side-effect of retrograde ejaculation; though it must be said that retrograde ejaculation can occur even after a laser prostatectomy due to laser damage to the bladder neck mechanism, and the catheter may need to stay *in situ* for some weeks after therapy. In addition, some patients complain of marked dysuria for many weeks after this procedure.

In the final analysis, a TURP is likely to result in a better outcome than any other alternatitve treatment, such as laser prostatectomy. Additionally, while the PSA value of 9.3 ng/mg may be due to retention and catheterization alone, it also raises the possibility of prostate cancer. Another advantage of treating this patient with a TURP is that the 'chippings' that result from this procedure would enable a histological diagnosis of prostate cancer to be excluded.

Case 9: Prostatism, cardiovascular co-morbidity

A 66-year-old retired man presents complaining of increased frequency of micturition by night and day, and of a long-standing reduction of the force of his urinary stream. He is known to have angina and has some degree of cardiac failure leading to treatment with a diuretic in the form of frusemide, 40 mg/day. He has been aware that his urinary symptoms have deteriorated since the diuretic was started, and he therefore avoids his medication in the morning if he plans to go outside the house. On examination, he is not in cardiac failure and the bladder is impalpable. On rectal examination, the prostate was asymmetrically enlarged, but smooth, and did not feel hard. His PSA was 10.2 ng/ml. How should this problem be dealt with?

Family practitioner. This case would be consistent with a patient with BPH; the raised PSA probably reflects the considerable benign enlargement of the gland. Referral, however, should be considered for two reasons:

- to confirm that the raised PSA was a result of benign rather than malignant disease
- because the patient's prostatic symptoms are interfering with the efficiency of therapy for his cardiac failure.

Medical therapy with finasteride would be a possibility if the results of transrectal biopsy confirmed the diagnosis of BPH, but the patient should be warned that the onset of symptom relief may take some months. Alpha blocker therapy is not advisable because it sometimes masks the symptoms of cardiac failure, though it does not cause deterioration in cardiovascular function.

Urologist. Yes, even if the prostate felt benign on DRE, with a PSA over 10 ng/ml, TRUS and a biopsy should be undertaken to confirm a diagnosis of BPH before deciding on management. Assuming that the

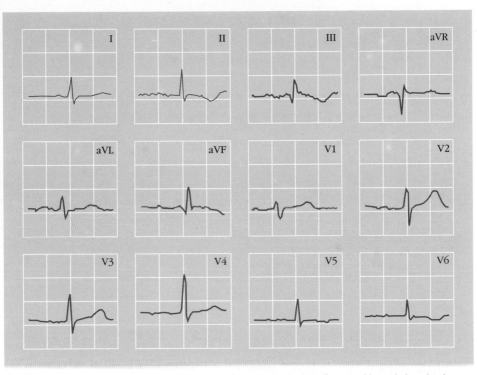

This ECG suggests ischaemia as there is T wave inversion in the inferior and lateral chest leads.

biopsies all showed BPH, then this patient would probably be best managed by TURP for rapid and complete relief of outflow obstruction. That is, of course, providing the cardiologists were happy that his mild heart failure and history of angina did not pose an undue risk during the anaesthesia – epidural or light general – necessary for TURP.

Case 10: Nocturia, normal flow

A 74-year-old man presents mainly with symptoms of nocturia. According to him, his urinary stream is quite normal, but he does admit to drinking quite large quantities of tea and beer in the evenings. What advice would you give him?

Family practitioner. Ask the 'three questions' and, in this case, positive answers on both nocturia and bother factor can be expected. His IPSS score would probably be above 8. DRE might reveal some mild benign enlargement of the prostate, but the point to remember here is that prostate size does not correlate with the presence or absence of obstruction. As the patient is reporting a normal urinary stream, his symptoms may well be based on a high fluid intake in the evenings producing nocturnal polyuria unassociated with outflow obstruction. However, patients do not always have a good perception of the normality of their stream, so obtain a PSA determination, a bladder ultrasound and an objective measurement of flow rate of this man.

Results

PSA	3.7 ng/ml
Maximum flow rate	16.3 ml/second
PVR volume	30 ml

Family practitioner. These results are reassuring; the prostate appears to be benign, and there is little to suggest significant bladder outflow obstruction. This patient might do quite well with simple counselling about reducing fluid intake in the evening. Polyuria in elderly patients may be unrelated to outflow obstruction and does not always indicate prostatic troubles. Careful examination of his cardiac and respiratory systems is therefore necessary, in addition to an MSU, U&E, creatinine and urine analysis for glycosuria.

Urologist. This patient complains of nocturia, but does not have any restriction of voiding. In addition, his flow rate is normal both subjectively and objectively, and his PVR is very low. There is nothing here to suggest that he is obstructed. The purists might suggest that he should have a full urodynamic assessment in order to exclude obstruction, but this may be considered excessively invasive by many urologists. Nocturia can be an extremely 'bothersome' symptom, but it may be caused by many other conditions apart from BPH. Particularly if nocturia is an isolated symptom, cardiac, renal and hepatic causes should be ruled out.

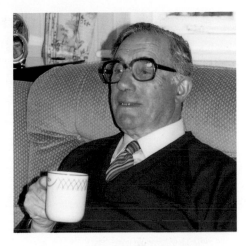

This patient's symptoms of nocturia are largely self-inflicted as a result of excessive drinking in the evening. Stopping this habit should be sufficient. If the patient still complains of symptoms and his flow rate is quite normal, then there are two lines of therapy that one might employ.

■ Firstly, an anticholinergic agent, such as oxybutynin, 5 mg, at night could be prescribed to try to inhibit unstable detrusor contractions, though this is not always effective in these patients.

■ The second and more reliable option is the use of an antidiuretic hormone analogue, such as 1-deamino-8-D-arginine vasopressin (DDAVP), which is very effective in reducing nocturia and can be administered in tablet form or by intranasal spray. Some patients with urinary frequency occasionally take this treatment during the day in situations when urinary frequency might be socially embarrassing.

Case 11: Perineal discomfort, dysuria, malaise

A 43-year-old man presents with a long-standing history of perineal discomfort associated with intermittent dysuria and a feeling of general malaise. On examination his prostate feels rather indurated, and is markedly tender on palpation bilaterally, but is not enlarged.

Family practitioner. This history would fit with a diagnosis of chronic prostatitis and, really, the question is whether it is bacterial or abacterial. Undertake a DRE and ask for a urine sample, both before the examination and after, to see whether massaging prostatic fluid into the urethra results in a positive culture of expressed prostatic secretions (EPS). Also check the PSA level. These patients are usually excessively anxious and sometimes do need referring on for specialist investigations, particularly TRUS with colour Doppler imaging. In addition, the kidneys should be imaged by ultrasound.

Results

MSU	Negative
Prostate massage specimen	WBC +++
Culture	Negative
Maximum flow rate	15.5 ml/second
PSA	0.8 ng/ml
TRUS	Diffuse hypervascularity of the peripheral zone with abnormal engorgement of the periprostatic veins

Urologist. The criteria for diagnosing chronic prostatitis have been described in detail. Without prostatic massage and analysis of prostatic secretions, it is a rather difficult condition to diagnose. It can be confused with several ill-defined maladies, such as prostatodynia, which present in a similar manner. Reassurance is important, and this

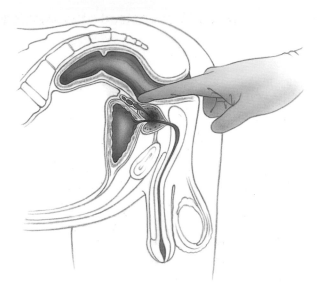

Massaging the prostate.
Prostatic secretions can be
massaged into the urethra and
collected for culture and
sensitivity studies.

may require that the full panoply of investigations be performed. In the absence of bacteria on prostatic massage, antibiotics play only a placebo role and do not have a specific therapeutic function. The use of many compounds in this symptom complex have been looked at only in open non-randomized studies, which do not fulfil statistical evaluation. Microwave thermotherapy is also probably only of placebo value in this condition. Non-steroidal anti inflammatory analgesics, such as ibuprofen and diclofenac, either orally or as a suppository, may be effective.

It has recently been suggested that the use of an alpha blocker to relax the bladder neck and improve the flow rate on these patients can be useful, but there are no controlled data to confirm this and no therapy is very effective. The symptoms tend to wax and wane. If pain in the perineum is the predominant symptom, it is sometimes helpful to refer patients to an expert in chronic pain. It is also worth rechecking the cultures with a formal lower tract localization test (i.e. massage of the prostate to obtain secretions and collection of divided specimens of urine) to be certain that there is no infection within the prostate.

Shared care for prostatic diseases

Case 12: Asymptomatic, positive family history

A middle-aged man who is asymptomatic, but has a family history of prostate cancer, has noted the recent publicity surrounding this disease and presents asking for a prostate check-up. On examination, his prostate feels of normal size with no areas of induration, but his PSA level is 6.3 ng/ml. How would you deal with this situation?

Family practitioner. This is an increasingly common scenario. The two warning signs in this case are the family history of prostate cancer and elevated PSA. Ask how old the patient's relative was when he developed prostate cancer, and how close a relative he was. The PSA is only mildly elevated, but in a middle-aged man with an apparently normal prostate, this could indicate the presence of a tumour. In view of his PSA and family history, this patient should be referred to a urologist for TRUS and biopsy.

Results

TRUS	Revealed an abnormal hypo-echoic area in the left transition zone with hypervascularity on colour Doppler imaging. Biopsy confirmed the presence of a well-differentiated adenocarcinoma of the prostate, Gleason grade 3

Urologist. Cases with biopsy-proven adenocarcinoma of the prostate are now presenting earlier in many countries because of:
- increased public awareness
- the availability of PSA determinations
- the enhanced ability to biopsy the prostate using TRUS.

A patient with a family history of prostate cancer is at considerable risk of developing prostate cancer, and should be screened carefully. This is an absolute indication for referral to a urologist, who should

164

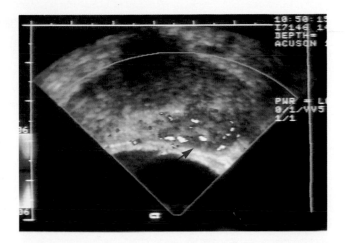

Colour Doppler of patient with prostate cancer showing a focal increase in blood flow in the tumour area.

perform a DRE and PSA, and if any doubt exists as to the interpretation of the results, a TRUS-guided prostate biopsy. This should, in the event of a negative survey, be repeated on a yearly basis. The finding of a PSA of 6.3 ng/ml further increases the index of suspicion and a sextant prostatic biopsy under TRUS control should be undertaken. If the biopsies are positive, the urologist should discuss with the patient the treatment options of radical prostatectomy or radical radiotherapy.

Case 13: Adenocarcinoma revealed by TURP

A 70-year-old man has recently presented in the Accident and Emergency Department with acute retention and has subsequently undergone TURP. Histology reveals BPH in most chippings, but several chips show the presence of well-differentiated adenocarcinoma of the prostate. The patient comes back to discuss these results with his family practitioner.

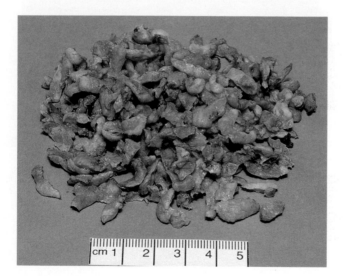

Histological examination of chips from TURP may reveal malignancy.

Family practitioner. Explain to the patient the process of TURP and how chippings are sent for pathological analysis. Tell him that the presence of adenocarcinoma of the prostate in two chippings may or may not be significant, but further analysis may be necessary by a urologist. Refer him to the urologist who performed the original surgery.

Urologist. In patients over 70 years of age, we would probably elect for external beam irradiation with careful PSA follow-up. If the conservative option of observation only was adopted in this patient's case, we would suggest 3-monthly PSA determinations, together with a TRUS and biopsy of the residual peripheral zone tissue at 3–6 months after TURP to exclude significant volume residual prostate cancer.

If the PSA increased by more than 20% over 1 year (or more than 0.75 ng/ml in absolute terms), or transrectal biopsies revealed the presence of residual cancer in the younger, fitter patient, more active therapy would be considered. This is defined as a T1a cancer of the prostate. Some studies show that in a healthy patient with a reasonable life expectancy of more than 10 years, definitive treatment should be suggested. TURP is not a satisfactory method of diagnosing prostatic cancer; many studies have shown that even in this situation a more extensive and more significant peripheral zone cancer can be missed. TURP will remove only the transition zone cancers whereas the more significant cancers occur in the peripheral zone, and these may be present in association with transition zone cancers.

Case 14: TURP and sexual concerns

A man aged 62 has seen the urologist and has been put on the waiting list for TURP. He asked his family practitioner what sexual problems could arise from this procedure.

Family practitioner. Patient awareness has increased considerably over the last few years and time needs to be set aside to discuss the sequelae of surgical procedures more fully. Postoperative sexual problems may cause patients and their partners considerable anxiety – matters which they often find difficult to discuss.

Prostatectomy, whether performed via the transurethral route or retropubic route, interferes with the bladder neck and results in failure of occlusion at the time of ejaculation. This causes retrograde ejaculation and therefore the patient is rendered sterile. There is often anxiety about the possible effects of retrograde ejaculation and the patient needs to be reassured that this is not harmful. It may be helpful to explain that, although sterility is universal, impotence is a rare complication of prostatectomy. This procedure is normally performed in an age group where sexual activity is already decreasing and any surgical procedure or major illness may cause impotence.

In the case of TURP, impotence may occasionally be caused by the heat generated in the region of the prostatic capsule as a result of resection and coagulation using diathermy. This generation of heat may damage the prostatic nerve plexus through which the corpora cavernosa and corpus spongiosum derive their nerve supply. However, impotence occurs in less than 10–16% of patients undergoing this procedure.

Urologist. Impotence is a strongly age-related disorder, and many cases that occur after TURP are probably incidental and not the result of surgery. A number of effective forms of treatment are now available for men with this problem. Oral agents are of limited value, although yohimbine, an alpha-2 adrenoceptor blocker, has been reported to

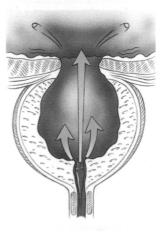

Retrograde ejaculation. After transurethral resection of the prostate (TURP), semen passes retrogradely into the bladder at the time of orgasm because of the loss of the bladder neck sphincter mechanism.

help some men with psychogenic impotence. Intracavernous pharmacotherapy with papaverine and phentolamine or prostaglandin E_1, is often effective, but carries a small but significant risk of inducing priapism. Vacuum devices and inflatable penile prostheses are two further treatment options.

Case 15: TURP and complication concerns

A man aged 60 years presents to his family practitioner for advice, having heard stories from some of his friends about complications of TURP, and asks whether he can have the operation performed abdominally to avoid the pain and bleeding he has been told about.

Family practitioner. Advise this patient that retropubic or transvesical prostatectomy has largely been replaced over the last 40 years with endoscopic resection, and now over 90% of prostatic surgery is carried out endoscopically through a resectoscope. These instruments have improved considerably over the years and even very large benign glands can be dealt with in this manner.

TURP has considerable advantages over open prostatectomy. It can be carried out under a spinal or epidural anaesthetic, there is no abdominal incision to cause complications with breathing or mobilization, and the hospital stay is much shorter. If the gland is extremely large and the risk of blood loss is considerable, or if there is an associated bladder stone or diverticulum which requires treatment, then the retropubic approach may be more appropriate.

In general, prostatectomy by the transurethral route significantly reduces the incidence of postoperative complications. Early mobility reduces the risk of respiratory and thrombo-embolic complications, and only a small percentage of patients will require postoperative transfusion.

With early discharge from hospital, family practitioners may see bleeding from the prostatic cavity in the early postoperative period, and obstruction by blood clot may require bladder wash-outs and possibly recatheterization. Urinary infection may cause troublesome postoperative dysuria and frequency, but these symptoms respond rapidly to antibiotics.

A rare, but serious, complication in the early postoperative period is the transurethral resection syndrome. This is the result of absorption of irrigating fluid into the circulation. The fluid overload may produce pulmonary oedema and the glycine, which is metabolized to ammonia, may cause confusion and even transient blindness.

There may, of course, be the need for a further operation, and estimates vary from 10–20% over a 10-year period. This may be necessary because of recurrent obstructive symptoms caused by further adenomatous deterioration in urine flow or urethral stricture caused by endoscopy. The incidence of urethral stricture is probably only 1–5%.

Finally, it is important to inform patients that TURP does not preclude the development of prostate cancer in the residual prostatic tissue at a later date.

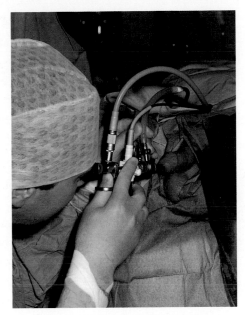

A transurethral resection of the prostate (TURP) in progress.

Case 16: Complementary medicine enquiries

A man aged 58 years attends the surgery. He is anxious to avoid prostate surgery and is not willing to try medical treatments. He asks your advice about what alternative and complementary medicines are available for his prostatic symptoms.

Family practitioner. BPH is a variable condition and the severity of the symptoms may fluctuate from week to week. This situation makes complementary medicine difficult to evaluate. There is, however, some commonsense advice that may be offered to this patient. A healthy diet and life-style should be encouraged with little or no alcohol or tobacco. The diet should contain foods that are high in fibre, low in cholesterol and saturated fats, and include plenty of fresh fruit and vegetables. Constipation should be avoided, and it is probably best to avoid spicy foods, coffee and strong tea, as these substances can increase bladder irritability.

Homoeopathy and plant extracts are widely used in Europe, and these treatments are claimed to improve prostatic symptoms by influencing both the size of the gland and the state of muscle tone at the bladder neck. It is also asserted that the irritability of the

---

General dietary advice

- Lose excess weight
- Low-fat diet
- Reduce saturated fats, especially red meat
- Increase unrefined carbohydrates, fibre and fish
- Minimum of five portions of fresh fruit or vegetables every day

obstructed bladder can be improved, but there are almost no placebo-controlled data to support this.

Medicines commonly available include extracts derived from stinging nettle root, golden rod flowers and the fruit of the saw palmetto. Such treatments have been marketed in Europe, particularly in France, Italy and West Germany, and the pills are available without prescription in most pharmacies in France.

Remedies containing zinc have been advocated over the last few years and, although zinc is found in high concentrations in the prostate gland in the seminal fluid, the function of this mineral is poorly understood. It has never been shown that the addition of an oral zinc supplement will prevent or treat any form of prostate disease or condition.

In all probability plant extracts are merely an expensive way of administering placebo. Before trying any of these remedies, the patient should certainly be advised to seek medical advice and have any necessary examinations and investigations.

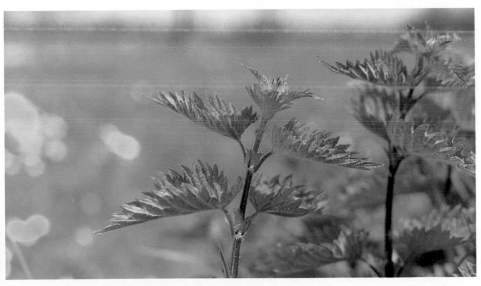

Louise Walsh

Case 17: Very elderly patient, severe prostatism

An 89-year-old gentleman who is mentally alert presents with severe prostatism. He is getting up six times in the night and has a very poor urinary flow. What would you advise?

Family practitioner: Very elderly patients, often with severe symptoms, inevitably have some age-related co-morbidity and are often disturbed by anything that disrupts their normal routine. Perform a full physical examination including a DRE. Measurement of PSA is not necessary because the result will not affect management. Providing the bladder is impalpable and creatinine is normal, consider medical therapy with either an alpha blocker using careful dose titration, or a 5-alpha-reductase inhibitor. Monitor the patient closely to evaluate his symptom response with IPSS and, if possible, flow rate determinations.

Results

MSU	Negative
Creatinine	Normal
PSA	Not requested
Maximum flow rate	8.5 ml/second
ECG	Severe ischaemia
IPSS	27

Urologist: Very elderly patients tolerate hospitalization and general anaesthesia poorly. Although this man is extremely symptomatic and probably severely obstructed, there is a good case for medical management here. However, if chronic or acute urinary retention were to develop, then an interventional procedure may become necessary. An alternative to a TURP might be the use of an intraprostatic stent which could be inserted under local anaesthetic. Stents have been shown to relieve obstruction effectively, but their long-term safety and efficacy is still unknown.

Index